Department of Veterans Affairs
Health Services Research & Development Service | Evidence-based Synthesis Program

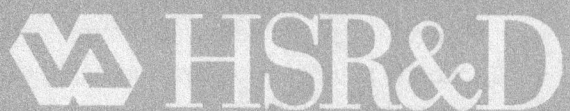

Systematic Review of Women Veterans Health Research 2004-2008

October 2010

Prepared for:
Department of Veterans Affairs
Veterans Health Administration
Health Services Research & Development Service
Washington, DC 20420

Prepared by:
Evidence-based Synthesis Program (ESP) Center
West Los Angeles VA Medical Center
Los Angeles, CA
Paul G. Shekelle, MD, PhD, Director

Investigators:
Principal Investigator:
Bevanne Bean-Mayberry, MD, MHS

Co-Investigators:
Christine Huang, MD
Fatma Batuman, MD
Caroline Goldzweig, MD, MSPH
Donna L. Washington, MD, MPH
Elizabeth M. Yano, PhD, MSPH

Research Associate:
Isomi M. Miake-Lye, BA

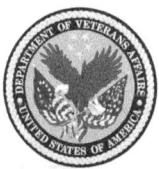

PREFACE

HSR&D's Evidence-based Synthesis Program (ESP) was established to provide timely and accurate syntheses of targeted healthcare topics of particular importance to VA managers and policymakers, as they work to improve the health and healthcare of Veterans. The ESP disseminates these reports throughout VA.

HSR&D provides funding for four ESP Centers and each Center has an active VA affiliation. The ESP Centers generate evidence syntheses on important clinical practice topics, and these reports help:

- develop clinical policies informed by evidence,
- the implementation of effective services to improve patient outcomes and to support VA clinical practice guidelines and performance measures, and
- set the direction for future research to address gaps in clinical knowledge.

In 2009, an ESP Coordinating Center was created to expand the capacity of HSR&D Central Office and the four ESP sites by developing and maintaining program processes. In addition, the Center established a Steering Committee comprised of HSR&D field-based investigators, VA Patient Care Services, Office of Quality and Performance, and VISN Clinical Management Officers. The Steering Committee provides program oversight and guides strategic planning, coordinates dissemination activities, and develops collaborations with VA leadership to identify new ESP topics of importance to Veterans and the VA healthcare system.

Comments on this evidence report are welcome and can be sent to Nicole Floyd, ESP Coordinating Center Program Manager, at nicole.floyd@va.gov.

Recommended citation:
Bean-Mayberry B, Batuman F, Huang C, Goldzweig CL, Washington DL, Yano EM, Miake-Lye I, Shekelle PG. Systematic Review of Women Veterans Health Research 2004-2008. VA-ESP Project #05-226; 2010

TABLE OF CONTENTS

EXECUTIVE SUMMARY

BACKGROUND

The body of literature dedicated to women veterans' health and health care issues has grown significantly since the publication of one previous systematic review focused on women veterans[1]. To address the growing demand and potential needs of women veterans in the Department of Veterans Affairs (VA) Healthcare System, this project sought to assess the state of women veterans' health research and stratify the literature into domains relevant for VA research and policy.

Because of the broad survey nature of this synthesis, no key questions were developed.

METHODS

We conducted a systematic review of the scientific literature on women veterans' health and health care published from 2004 to 2008. Articles were identified by searching multiple scientific databases, and supplemented through direct contact with Department of Defense, VA and other experts in the field. Article titles were screened by the whole synthesis team, and those articles deemed potentially relevant to the review were each independently evaluated by two of three reviewers (BB, CH, FB) using a standard screening form. Disagreements in assessment were resolved by consensus with input from at least one senior member of the research team. Articles were considered for inclusion if the study related to U.S. veterans or military personnel and met at least one of the following three criteria: (a) included women veterans, compared men and women, or analyzed women separately; (b) involved active duty military women and a health condition or functional status that requires medical attention; or (c) were relevant to women veterans' health in VA or how VA care is delivered to women. We excluded articles that were non-systematic reviews, editorials, commentaries or of unclear study design. Because of the heterogeneity of the studies, no formal meta-analysis could be performed. Articles were classified according to subject category and narratively summarized in evidence tables.

RESULTS

We retrieved 675 articles, of which 380 were unique and passed a title screen for relevance. Of these, 185 articles were rejected because the inclusion criteria were not met: 48 did not relate to U.S. veterans or military personnel; 106 failed to meet at least one of the other three inclusion criteria; 31 articles were excluded because the study design was not appropriate (non-systematic reviews, editorials, commentaries, and unclear designs). The remaining 195 articles were categorized by study design, funding source, period of military service (if specified) of study subjects, research topic area, and health conditions addressed.

Nearly 60 percent of studies were supported by VA funds. We identified 85 articles focused on psychiatry and mental health issues, across the broad categories of PTSD, general mental health, trauma (including military sexual trauma) and other conditions. The next largest set of articles focused on quality of care (54); access and utilization (48); post-deployment health issues, especially related to OEF/OIF veterans (33); and organizational research (7). Categories were not mutually exclusive.

CONCLUSIONS

The literature on women veterans has increased substantially. The baseline review covering the more than two decades between 1978 and 2004 included 182 articles. The updated review covering the 5-year period 2004 to 2008 included 195 articles. Therefore, more women veterans health articles have been published in the past 5 years than in the 23 years before that.

Consistent with the previous systematic review, most VA women's health research continues to be observational. However, more articles are shifting from a descriptive to an analytical focus (e.g., determinants of care or health), and there has been a modest increase in the number of clinical trials—two in the baseline review, 5 in this update review.

Although the focus on mental health among women in the military and women veterans remains high, with a continuing emphasis on PTSD and MST, important new work has been published on prevalence of mental health conditions in different settings and for different subgroups and on non-trauma-related mental health problems (e.g., depression, serious mental illness). Emphasis on access, utilization, and quality of care for women veterans has increased, as has a focus on post-deployment health. These topics were identified in the baseline review as vital gaps in the literature and map to VA research priorities. Therefore, the past 5 years have seen substantial alignment between priority areas for women veterans' health research and the research topics being pursued.

INTRODUCTION

BACKGROUND

Women are playing an ever increasing role in the US military, representing about 15% of active military personnel, 17% of reserve and National Guard forces, and 20% of new military recruits. Concurrently, women are one of the fastest growing groups of new users in the Department of Veterans Affairs (VA) Healthcare System, with particularly high rates of utilization among veterans of Operation Enduring Freedom (OEF) and Operation Iraqi Freedom (OIF). Of the more than 100,000 OEF/OIF women veterans, over 44% have enrolled in the VA system for health care[2]. Thus, women veterans represent an integral part of the veteran community.

Women's military experiences and responses to their military experiences are often distinct from those of men, and these differences can affect both their health status and their health care needs as active duty personnel and as veterans. This, together with the rise in the number of women veterans in the VA system, calls for increased understanding of women veteran health issues and areas of potential knowledge deficit in order to guide VA care and VA research efforts. The body of research literature dedicated to women veterans and women's military health and health care issues has significantly grown and expanded in size and scope since the publication of the first systematic review of women veterans research[1]. This project updated that review by examining the literature on women veterans' health and health care from 2004 to 2008.

METHODS

TOPIC DEVELOPMENT

This project was nominated by Linda Lipson, HSR&D Equity Portfolio Manager, and the Office of Women's Health.

Because of the broad survey nature of this synthesis, no key questions were developed.

SEARCH STRATEGY

We searched MEDLINE/PubMed, PsycINFO, WorldCat and Web of Science for potentially relevant articles related to women veteran and military health published between January 2004 and September 2008. For each database search, we used the medical subject heading (MeSH) terms *women* and *veterans* to search for relevant literature. We supplemented this search by contacting other sources with expertise in the area of women veteran and military health. The Department of Defense Health Affairs Division provided access to bibliographical reports on general deployment and mental health issues in Operation Enduring Freedom and Operation Iraqi Freedom (OEF/OIF) military personnel from 2002 through 2007[3]. We received additional articles from a direct request to experts in the field via a VA research list service and personal contact with approximately 15 VA women's health researchers. We also identified additional articles by reviewing bibliographies from articles identified through our search. The search strategy is listed in Appendix 4.

STUDY SELECTION

All titles identified through our search were screened for relevance by the members of the team. Each article deemed potentially relevant was reviewed by two physician reviewers with backgrounds in women's health working independently (BB, FB, CH) using a standardized, one page screening form (Appendix 1) and these assessments were compared and reconciled. Disagreements in ratings were resolved through consensus resolution with the help of at least one senior member of the review team. To be included, articles had to meet criteria (a), plus at least one of criteria (b), (c), or (d). The criteria were: (a) study relates to U.S. veterans or military personnel; (b) study includes women veterans, compares men and women, or analyzes women separately; (c) study involves active duty military and involves a health condition or functional status that requires medical intervention; and (d) topic is relevant to VA healthcare or to how VA care is delivered to women (Appendix 3). An article was excluded if it was defined as a non-systematic review, editorial, commentary, or an unclear publication type.

DATA ABSTRACTION

After the initial screening process, articles meeting inclusion criteria were further evaluated and abstracted using a structured abstract form (Appendix 2). The following data were abstracted: year(s) of study or sampling timeframe; purpose of study, outcomes reported; study population description; whether the article was women-focused or had women as a subset population, or neither; brief summary of methods; and main findings. Additional data collected covered basic information about each article: study design, sample size (both female and male), study setting (from where the study population was drawn), military period of service studied (if specified), women's health research topic area, specific condition(s) studied and study funding.

QUALITY ASSESSMENT

For the few clinical trials identified, we used Jadad criteria for quality assessment[4]. For the descriptive studies, which are by far the largest number of studies, no simple standardized assessment of quality exists, and therefore, a quality assessment protocol is not included in this review.

DATA SYNTHESIS

We identified 5 key focus areas for the Women's Health Evidence Synthesis Project, using high priority areas identified by the 2004 review by Goldzweig and associates[1], and the VA Health Services Research and Development Service (HSR&D) funding priorities. The areas were the following:

- Deployment and post-deployment health
- Organizational research
- Quality of care
- Access to care and utilization
- Psychiatric conditions.

Below we briefly describe the relationship between these categories and those in the baseline review. We then summarize the findings of articles in each of area and highlight their significance.

CROSS WALK BETWEEN BASELINE REVIEW AND UPDATED REVIEW

The baseline review grouped the available literature into four categories; the update review groups literature into 5 categories, reflecting the growth in the scientific literature in the areas of access, utilization, and quality of care. Figure 1 shows the cross walk between the categories for each review and provides explanatory notes.

Figure 1 Category Cross Walk

Categories in updated review (2004 – 2008)	Categories in baseline review (1978 - 2004)	Comments
Deployment and post-deployment health	Stress of military life	A substantial body of work now focuses on OEF/OIF veterans as well as on women's health issues in the theatre
Organizational research	Health services research	Formerly included in the general health services research category. More focused literature has emerged examining how organizational factors affect women's health care delivery environment and the overall practice environment
Quality of care	Health services research	The literature on quality of care is now substantially expanded, including patient perceptions of quality and satisfaction and general quality of care processes and outcomes
Access/utilization	Health services research; Health and performance of military or VA women	The new category reflects the volume of work on determinants of access/ utilization especially for special cohorts of veterans
Psychiatric conditions	Psychiatric conditions; Health and performance of military or VA women	New work describes prevalence of mental health conditions in different settings and for different subgroups and addresses non-trauma related health problems

PEER REVIEW

A draft version of this report was sent to seven peer reviewers, of which five responded. Their comments and our responses are presented in Appendix 10.

RESULTS

LITERATURE FLOW

Our search identified 675 titles of potential relevance. Of these titles, 118 were duplicate references to a study, 151 were rejected as not being relevant to the topic, and 26 could not be retrieved. Of the remaining 380 articles that were evaluated as full-text articles by at least two physician reviewers independently, 154 were rejected because they did not meet our inclusion criteria; 48 did not relate to U.S. veterans or military personnel; and 106 failed to meet at least one of the following additional criteria. Thirty-one articles were excluded because the study design was not appropriate: 4 articles were non-systematic reviews, 22 were editorials or commentaries, and 5 articles had unclear design.

Further data abstraction was performed on the remaining 195 articles, and all were categorized into the following 5 areas, which were not mutually exclusive: deployment and post-deployment health issues (n=33); organizational research (n=7); quality of care (n=54); access and utilization (n=48); and psychiatric conditions (n=85) (See Figure 2).

Figure 2 Literature Flow

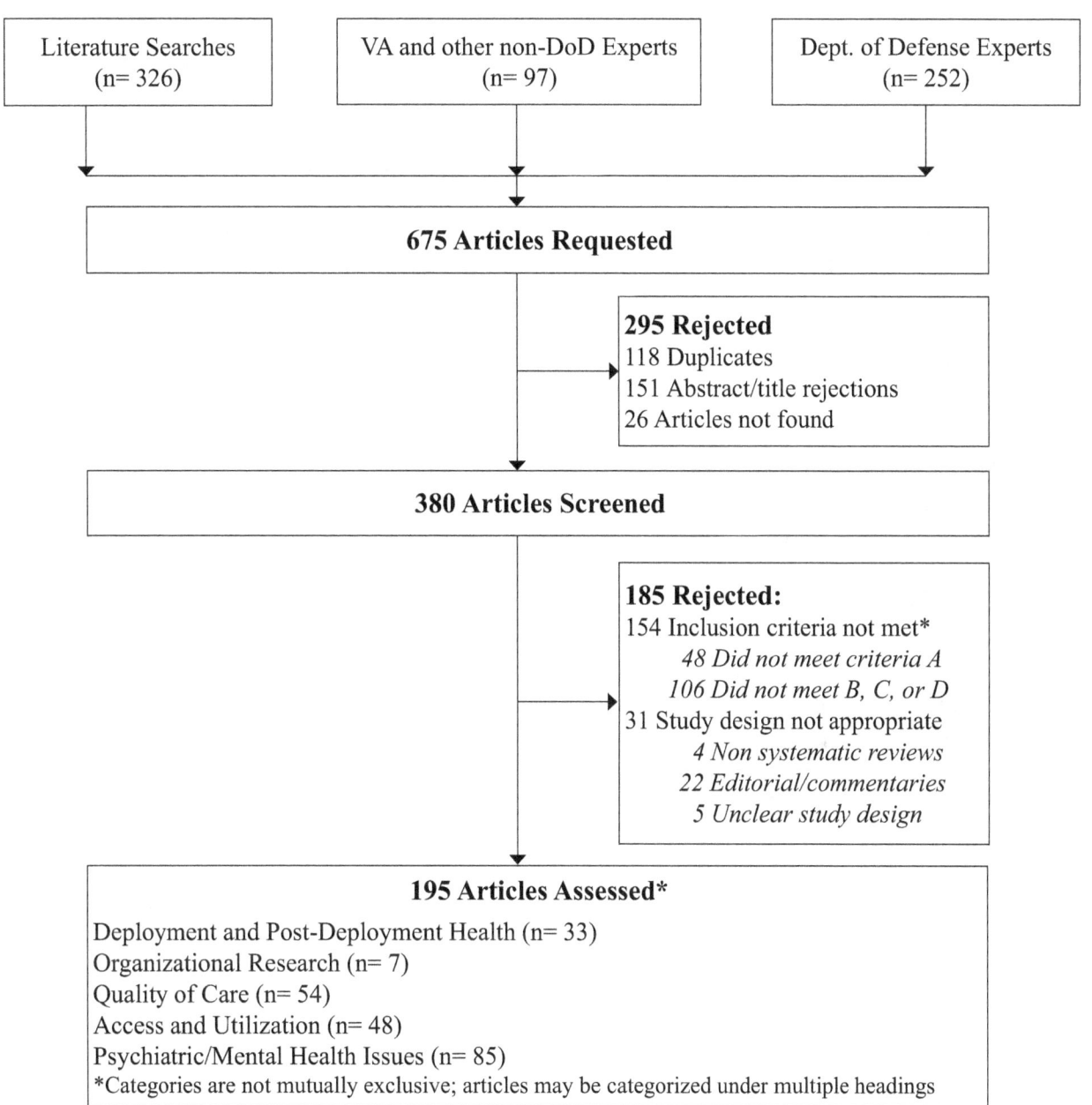

| Literature Searches (n= 326) | VA and other non-DoD Experts (n= 97) | Dept. of Defense Experts (n= 252) |

675 Articles Requested

295 Rejected
118 Duplicates
151 Abstract/title rejections
26 Articles not found

380 Articles Screened

185 Rejected:
154 Inclusion criteria not met*
   48 Did not meet criteria A
   106 Did not meet B, C, or D
31 Study design not appropriate
   4 Non systematic reviews
   22 Editorial/commentaries
   5 Unclear study design

195 Articles Assessed*

Deployment and Post-Deployment Health (n= 33)
Organizational Research (n= 7)
Quality of Care (n= 54)
Access and Utilization (n= 48)
Psychiatric/Mental Health Issues (n= 85)
*Categories are not mutually exclusive; articles may be categorized under multiple headings

DESCRIPTION OF EVIDENCE

As in the baseline systematic review[1], the majority of articles discussed observational or descriptive studies. Nearly half of the research articles focused on psychiatric issues (e.g., screening for mental health conditions or for post traumatic stress disorder (PTSD).

Only five studies were identified as experimental studies or clinical trials. Of these, three focused on women veterans or military personnel with PTSD diagnosis or symptoms[5-7], one on VA employees' perceptions about women veterans[8] and one on improving mammography screening among women veterans[9]. Compared to the initial systematic review, these trials highlight a few key advances in methods by including the first VA multi-site randomized controlled trial on women veterans using the cooperative study program, and a moderately large sized mental health patient sample (N=284)[6].

Due to the broad scope of research contained in this report, each study has to be interpreted subject to its own limitations, and it is not feasible to include all the caveats and constraints within this document. Before citing specific findings, the reader should refer to the source article to understand the context of the research methods and findings.

DEPLOYMENT AND POST-DEPLOYMENT HEALTH

Thirty-three articles covered deployment and post deployment-health issues, with the majority of studies (n=23) addressing health issues specific to OEF/OIF veterans[10-32]. The OEF/OIF topics focused on mental health screenings, general women's deployment health issues, validation of the deployment risk and resilience inventory (DRRI), and psychiatric diagnoses associated with medical evacuation from the combat theatre. The remaining articles consisted of deployment studies in non-OEF/OIF cohorts (n=10)[33-42].

Studies Specific to OEF/OIF

Twenty-three studies addressed post-deployment health issues specific to OEF/OIF veterans; most focused on general mental health screening/utilization, PTSD symptoms, or access to services while deployed or upon return post-deployment.

Mental Health Screening and Utilization

The bulk of articles focused on mental health issues and OEF/OIF deployment. In this group (n=14), the majority of studies focused on mental health screening before, during, or after deployment among military personnel or recently returning veterans[10-13, 15, 17, 20-25, 27, 28]. Four themes are prominent in these studies: (1) high rates of screen positive PTSD symptoms (range 10-19%)[10, 11, 13, 15, 23, 28] or other mental health disorders[11, 12, 15, 17, 20-22, 24, 28] occur among OEF/OIF returning military women; (2) women in the military who recently returned from OEF/OIF deployments are disproportionately or more affected by symptoms of PTSD, symptoms of depression, other mental health issues or more likely referred for mental health care compared with men in the military who were recently deployed[11, 20, 22, 28]; (3) younger age and separated or divorced marital status tend to place military members at risk for more mental health symptoms[21, 22, 25]; and (4) a greater number of OIF deployments appears to be associated with screening positive for mental health problems[17, 20, 22].

PTSD Symptoms in OEF/OIF

Two studies assessed general assault history or Military Sexual Trauma (MST) history[10, 16]. The first by Smith and associates identified a doubled rate of new onset PTSD symptoms among combat military women (22% vs 10%) who had been exposed to assault prior to combat vs not, and also among military men (12% vs 6%)[10]. The second by Katz et al evaluated a small group of women (n=18) previously deployed who were referred for mental health care and compared their readjustments to civilian life and experiences in war compared with men. Over half the group (56%) were identified as having a MST history, based on a 3-item screen[16]. The two major study findings were that (1) of three types of events (MST, being injured, and witnessing others injured or killed), only MST was significantly related to the severity of clinical symptoms and difficulty with readjustment to civilian life, and (2) women who had MST had more symptoms and more difficulties with readjustment to civilian life than those without MST.

Access to Services

A salient finding by Seal and associates related to managing mental health symptoms and diagnoses was that mental health visits occurring within 90 days of screening were more likely to occur in veterans seen in VA community clinics versus the medical center (aOR 6.08; 95%CI 1.56, 23.6) or seen in any VA primary care clinic compared with other VA outpatient settings (aOR 19.4; 95%CI 1.30, 290)[24]. One small study captured potential barriers to mental health treatment reported by OIF National Guard soldiers, including stigma associated with seeking mental health treatment, pride, not being able to ask for help, and not being able to admit to having a problem[27].

Two additional studies analyzed the psychiatric diagnoses associated with medical evacuation from the theatre of combat[18, 19]. Stetz et al. analyzed the characteristics and diagnoses of medical evacuees from combat theatres during 2001-2003[18]. Women represented 16 and 18% of OIF and OEF evacuees respectively, and psychiatric diagnoses were the 2nd most common reason for evacuation from OEF and the 4th most common reason in OIF for the group overall. Rundell et al. found that psychiatric evacuees were more likely to be women, African-American or Hispanic, under the age of 31, and enlisted in the National Guard Reserve, as opposed to active duty military[19]. The most compelling finding was that women were overrepresented as psychiatric evacuees by a factor of 2.

A single study by Pierce on pregnant women[32] with recently deployed partners showed that these women often reported higher stress levels than those with homeland partners (39.6% and 24.2%; p<0.01). Regression analyses revealed that having a partner deployed, being active duty, advanced gestational age, and having >1child at home (OR 2.30, 95% CI 1.12-4.73) all predicted higher stress reporting. However, having a support person present was protective against stress (OR 0.40, 95% CI 0.20-0.78). These data included both military and nonmilitary pregnant women living on base and obtaining obstetric care at Naval Hospital.

General Deployment Health Issues

Two studies focused on military women in the field of duty[29, 30]. The Farley and colleagues document the number of gynecologic visits to a far forward combat support hospital at Bagram Air Force Base in Afghanistan compared with transport out of the regional area to Germany and the average number of work hours lost[29]. Over 90% of women (57 of 62) were seen in theatre at the Air Force Combat Support Hospital (CSH). Most patients had abnormal cervical cytology and colposcopies; other diagnoses included pregnancy, dysfunctional uterine bleeding and pelvic pain. The average work time loss during in theatre treatment was 6 woman-hours per patient compared with 216 hours per patient with travel to Germany. This paper underscores the benefits of providing far forward gynecology care (or gender-specific care) in the theatre of operations in order to maintain military readiness.

The second study by Thomson and colleagues anonymously surveyed women in the military deployed to Iraq or Kuwait for at least 3 months to assess their perceptions of health care delivery in OIF at the front line and aid stations[30]. Irregular bleeding (26%) and changes in hormonal contraception (23%) were the most common complaints among soldiers. Additionally, 21% of soldiers experienced some type of gynecological problem, and nearly one-half of patients (44%) did not meet the cervical cytology screening practice guidelines.

These studies highlighted the need to (1) complete routine gynecological screening at least 6 months before deployment to account for any abnormal results and allow for follow up, (2) educate non-gynecologic medical personnel on gender-specific issues, especially related to cycle control and contraception, and (3) provide at least a 3 month and preferably 6-12 month supply of hormonal contraception for women deployed. Each of these issues affects the military readiness of women soldiers.

Deployment Risk and Resilience Inventory

A single study by Vogt and associates validated 9 scales of the Deployment Risk and Resilience Inventory (DRRI) among a sample of OIF active duty soldiers who participated both before and after deployment[31]. In general, all DRRI scales demonstrated reasonable to excellent values for internal consistency and reliability (coefficient alpha or cronbach's alpha ranged from 0.77 to 0.90) suggesting that the item sets converged on a common construct. Only one construct had a lower cronbach's alpha (alpha = 0.55), and it was related to post deployment life stressors. Significant gender differences emerged for 5 of the DRRI scales. Men reported greater exposure to combat and aftermath of battle and more often reported being well prepared for deployment, and women reported greater perceived threat and less preparedness for battle compared with the men.

Other Studies

The remaining studies covered a sundry of topics ranging from environmental and physical health exposures reported by veterans (e.g., burning of trash and feces in OIF, genito-urinary concerns)[14], to case reports on the use of aripiprazole with sertraline or cognitive behavioral therapy for the treatment of PTSD symptoms such as sleep disorders in returning combat veterans[26].

General Deployment Issues - Non OEF/OIF

OEF/OIF deployment and mental health findings are described above in Studies Specific to OEF/OIF. The remaining ten deployment and mental health articles are not specific to the OEF/OIF cohorts[33-42]. A study on Bosnian peacekeeping veterans showed that longer deployments and first time deployments were associated with increased distress scores for male soldiers specifically; longer deployments did not show this effect in women veterans[33]. Among a sample of Vietnam veteran females, those who had a history of PTSD symptoms were susceptible to greater distress after the onset of Operation Desert Storm across all PTSD symptoms of re-experiencing, avoidance/numbing, and hyperarousal[37]. In contrast, risk of a mental health related hospitalization was lower among women in combat support occupations compared to women in non-combat support (HR0.64, 95% CI 0.53, 0.77) in a study occurring prior to the onset of OEF/OIF[35]. Among a mixed gender group of Gulf War I veterans, lower levels of social support resulted in increased depression symptoms for women, and increased levels of sexual harassment resulted in increased depression symptoms for men but not women suggesting that social support was a greater risk factor for depression in women and sexual harassment was a stronger risk factor for men[34]. Even in a small mixed gender case series of World War II veterans, 25% still had some PTSD symptoms 50 years after war[36]. The authors of this study suggest that studies of high functioning female and male veterans who have survived combat experiences and other trauma may be needed to provide more insight to veteran experiences and resiliency.

The baseline health status (physical and mental health component scores) of a large population-based military cohort is slightly more favorable than that of the same-age, same-sex U.S. general population, especially among older age groups, and also much higher than levels reported in VA populations presenting for care[38]. Deployment experiences were not associated with either decreased overall health status or mental well being[38, 39]. However, after adjustments for socio-demographics, deployment experience in SW Asia, Bosnia, or Kosovo (from 1998-2000), and deployment to the 1991 Gulf War, active-duty women health care specialists were significantly more likely to report witnessing death or trauma when compared to combat specialists[40]. In addition, Air Force women deployed to theatre during the Gulf War reported significantly more general as well as gender-specific health problems than did women deployed elsewhere[39]. Common health problems included: skin rash; cough; depression; unintentional weight loss; insomnia; and memory problems and a significant increase in gender-specific problems compared to women deployed elsewhere (e.g., abnormal pap, breast problems).

Two additional studies covered deployment related reproductive and pregnancy issues[41, 42]. The most prevalent gender-specific problems among an active duty sample (from Persian Gulf War) were problems during pregnancy (41%), urinary tract infection (34%), headache (33%), menstrual irregularities (32%) and abnormal Pap smear (27%)[42]. In this group, 76% reported using military health care, 41% used civilian health care, and only 3% reported using the VA. Overall, satisfaction ratings were higher for civilian care, and too few patients attended the VA to provide satisfaction ratings.

Another study[41] compared conceptions and pregnancy loss among Gulf War exposed conceptions and non-deployed conceptions among veterans and found similar outcomes. Separately, GW veteran postwar conceptions were at increased risk for ectopic pregnancies and spontaneous abortions, but the study was limited due to lack of information on risk factors for and documentation of fetal loss.

Summary

The large number of studies focused on the health issues of OEF/OIF soldiers reflects the growing participation of women in these conflicts. More than half of the OEF/OIF articles underscore the need to screen for PTSD and other mental health symptoms among recently returning soldiers who might have multiple risk factors. A key finding is that psychiatric diagnoses were common for both OEF and OIF evacuations, suggesting the need for DOD and VA to ensure that military personnel evacuated from the field for mental health issues receive ongoing care.

Two other salient issues arose in this section. First, both women and men with assault histories prior to combat had double the rates of new onset PTSD symptoms. Second, military readiness for women includes field access to gynecological services. These issues will be key for both DOD and VA in post-deployment health care settings.

ORGANIZATIONAL RESEARCH

The seven studies in this category all examined organizational characteristics of clinics delivering services to women in a national or regional sample of VA sites for primary care [43-49].

Services Available to Women

A national survey of VA facilities delivering primary care documented that 61% had established women's health clinics (WHC) for primary care; the main factor significantly related to the presence of WHCs was separate primary care leadership (OR 3.62, 95% CI 1.45-9.05)[43]. Three papers evaluating VA sites across the country serving 400 or more women veterans defined the presence of emergency services for women and the breadth and depth of gynecological services in the VA. Washington and colleagues assessed whether women's health care specialists for emergency gynecological problems or for emergency mental health conditions were available during and after clinic hours[46]. They found that while most sites had a specialist available for gynecologic and mental health emergencies during clinic hours, rates dropped for after-hour emergencies. Predictors of specialist availability were presence of a separate WHC for gynecological emergencies and lower local managed care penetration for mental health emergencies.

Cope and colleagues evaluated the availability of different forms of contraception in VA[47]. While 97% of VA sites provided hormonal contraception, only 60% of offered intrauterine devices (IUDs). Factors related to IUD service availability were hospital-based facility (in contrast to community-based outpatient clinic), on site gynecologist, and availability of a women's health clinician who trained other clinicians. Seelig and colleagues built on this work by assessing availability of gynecologic services across VA[44]. They found that availability of endometrial biopsy, IUD, infertility evaluation, infertility treatment, and general gynecologic surgery were directly related to routine availability of an Ob/Gyn physician.

Practice Environment

Hall et al. presented an assessment of organizational factors impacting the MST practice environment and perceived organizational support using key surveys of MST health providers in a VA geographical region[48]. Wide variability in the perception of organizational support existed among facilities even with a small sample size. Ethical conflicts, burnout, vicarious trauma experiences (i.e., from counseling), and isolation had negative correlations with perceived organizational support while workload, organizational culture, leadership, and MST resources were positively correlated with perceived organizational support.

Two studies focused on the organizational features associated with the adoption of women's health centers into VA sites[43, 49]. The first[43] examined primary care organizational features influencing the development of women's clinics in primary care (VAMCs or CBOCs) and found that nearly two-thirds of VAMCs had women's clinics (64%), but the only factor significantly associated with their presence was separate strong primary care leadership (OR 3.62, 95% CI 1.45, 9.05). Separately, Yano and colleagues[49] identified the degree to which VA medical centers had adopted women's clinics as an organizational innovation by comparing their structure and services to the 8 original Comprehensive Women's Health Centers (CWHCs) in VA. Gender specific service availability was comparable to the CWHCs with the exception of onsite mammography, osteoporosis assessment, and availability of separate mental health clinics[49]. While the general WHCs were less likely to have same gender providers, women's health training programs, separate space, or adequate privacy, they also were *less likely* to experience educational program closures or staffing losses.

The final study compared the original 8 VA Comprehensive Women's Health Centers with the Department of Health and Human Services (DHHS) National Centers of Excellence in Women's Health[45]. These prototype women's health centers had many parallel organizational characteristics (e.g., training or fellowship programs, quality monitoring activities, and extended hours or same gender providers) and uniformly provided preventive cancer screening, and general reproductive services. However, DHHS sites had more extensive reproductive care on site, and VA centers had more on-site mental health care.

Summary

Two issues are salient in this area. Presence of an Ob/Gyn physician in the VA or a separate gynecology or women's clinic in the VA improves the availability of IUD contraception, advanced gynecologic services, and emergency gynecologic services after hours. Separately, organizational culture and leadership showed positive associations with the practice environment for MST providers and with sites reporting separate women's clinics delivering primary care, indicating that key role of VA local leadership in women veteran care.

QUALITY OF CARE

Our summary of the quality of care literature on women veterans included fifty one studies that covered the following areas: patient perceptions of quality and ratings of satisfaction[50-58], general quality of care processes and outcomes[59-68], surgical outcomes[69-72], prescription medication issues[73-77], cardiovascular risk factors and health disparities[59, 60, 62, 63, 69, 70, 78-80], gender-specific and reproductive care[32, 41, 42, 81-91], other quality of care issues[92-98], and two clinical trials[8, 9].

Patient Perceptions of Quality and Satisfaction

Patient preferences in VA care among women veteran users and non-users were explored through a qualitative study by Washington and colleagues, which demonstrated knowledge gaps about VA eligibility and services[51]. These gaps included a general lack of information about VA eligibility and available services; nonusers often assumed that the VA did not provide women's health care. Separately, both users and nonusers identified the availability and accessibility of physicians and treatments, gender specific knowledge and sensitivity, and quality expertise and knowledge among the physicians/providers as expectations for their care. However, users and nonusers differed in perceptions of VA quality, and VA environment and quality concerns led many women to limit their VA use to women's clinics.

In a regional study of women veterans, Bean-Mayberry and associates examined patient race and primary care ratings in VA[50]. Race had no association with any of four primary care domains or with overall satisfaction with VA care. Separately, patients who reported that they received routine gynecological care from VA providers gave high ratings on preference for provider (OR 2.0, 95% CI 1.3, 3.1) and satisfaction (OR 1.6, 95% CI 1.2, 2.3).

Women's Clinics Versus Traditional Clinics

In a comparison of women veterans using women's clinics versus traditional primary care clinics, Bean-Mayberry et al. found that female veterans who were seen in the women's clinics were more likely to report excellent satisfaction compared with those seen in traditional clinics (p<.05, OR 1.42, 95% CI 1.00, 2.02)[52]. Similarly, for every domain in the original version of the Primary Care Satisfaction Survey for Women, patients seen in women's clinics were significantly more likely to report the highest satisfaction rating: getting care (OR 1.69, 95% CI 1.14, 2.49); privacy and comfort (OR 1.63, 95% CI 1.11, 2.39); communication (OR 1.66, 95% CI 1.16, 2.37); complete care (OR 1.69, 95% CI 1.17, 2.43); and follow up care (OR 1.70, 95% CI 1.16, 2.47).

Inpatient/Outpatient Satisfaction

Wright and associates compared patient satisfaction among male and female veterans in inpatient and outpatient settings in the VA nationally[53]. They found that in adjusted analyses, overall quality perceptions and most dimensions of satisfaction with outpatient care were not different for females compared with males. However, women were less satisfied than men for inpatient settings in multiple domains. Men reported higher scores for inpatient quality, after adjustment for transitions (68 vs. 65, p=0.0009), physical comfort (82 vs. 80, p=0.0003), involvement of family and friends (74 vs. 71, p=0.0024), courtesy (88 vs. 86, p=0.0001), coordination (77 vs. 74, p=0.0000), and access (80 vs. 76, p=0.0000).

Gender and Gynecological Services

Bean-Mayberry and colleagues determined whether the separate or combined effects of provider gender, gynecologic services from the provider, and women's clinic setting improved patient ratings of primary care[54]. Each combination was compared to a baseline of male provider, no gynecologic care from provider and no women's clinic setting. Having a female provider was significantly associated with the highest ratings for communication (OR 2.9, 95% CI 1.4, 5.8) and coordination (OR 3.7, 95% CI 1.5, 9.0). Male providers who provided gynecologic care or had patients enrolled in women's clinic had a higher rating of coordination (OR 3.0, 95% CI 1.2, 7.0) (compared with male providers who did not). Female providers who performed gynecological services also had significant positive associations in 3 of 4 domains: continuity (OR 4.0, 95% CI 1.8, 8.7); communication (OR 2.7, 95% CI 1.3, 5.5); and coordination (OR 2.8, 95% CI 1.1, 7.1). Similar findings occurred for patients who had all 3 factors (female provider, received gynecologic services, and used a women's clinic setting).

Fan and associates evaluated the relationship between continuity of care and satisfaction among women and men veterans in primary care at 7 medical centers using the Seattle-based Outpatient Satisfaction Questionnaire which has both a humanistic and organizational scale[57]. The humanistic scale measures satisfaction with communication skills and humanistic qualities of the providers, and the organizational scale measures satisfaction with the delivery of health care services. Higher patient reports of continuity of care were associated with higher patient satisfaction. Patients who reported always seeing the same provider had higher mean humanistic scores and mean satisfaction scores than those who rarely or never saw the same provider. Additionally, female patient gender and increasing age was associated with improved satisfaction and higher humanistic scores.

Mental Health

Two studies assessed the association of mental health with satisfaction in primary care[55, 58]. The first surveyed women in one VA healthcare system to identify the associations between satisfaction in general medical clinics and trauma-related mental health symptoms. The study found that women with *more* PTSD symptoms appeared to be more satisfied with their overall care and with their provider[55]. Separately, Desai and colleagues, evaluating VA patients with and without psychiatric illnesses who responded to a national VA satisfaction survey, found that patients with mental health diagnoses had lower satisfaction in outpatient primary care[58]. Dissatisfaction was associated with poorer perceptions of access to care and overall coordination of care.

Maternity Care

One study evaluated women's satisfaction with maternity care in 44 military hospitals and found that less than 50% of the respondents would recommend their hospital of care to family or friends due to a higher-than-average rate of problems with care[56]. Although this study had a fairly low response rate (41%), the data identify multiple quality and satisfaction issues: problem rates were significantly higher for these women compared with average Picker scores from patients nationwide. Military women reported worse ratings on satisfaction domains or items covering confidence and trust in provider, treatment with respect and dignity, involvement with medical decision-making, and coordination of care (p<.0001 for each). These experiences are directly related to maternity care in military hospitals; however, such experiences may affect expectations about potential VA health care after active duty.

General Quality of Care Prevention, Processes and Outcomes

Ten quality of care studies focused on general prevention and chronic disease processes[59-68].

One study, which focused on patterns of colorectal cancer screening in fiscal year 2002, noted that screening was most likely in patients aged 70-80 years. Factors associated with lower screening included: female gender; black race; lower income; infrequent primary care visits; and recent admission to a nursing home setting[61]. One salient clinical finding was that 41% of patients with a positive fecal occult blood test were not offered any type of colon examination within a 6-month window. Another study[66] explored the barriers, attitudes and preferences for colorectal cancer (CRC) screening by gender and found that female and male participants reported similar preferences for CRC screening mode, but women viewed the preparation for endoscopic procedures as a major barrier to screening while men did not. Women also expressed different fears from men (vulnerability vs. pain) and perceived CRC as a male disease thus feeling less vulnerable to CRC. These gender-specific barriers may help explain women's lower rate of screening for CRC. In a separate analyses examining flu vaccination by race among outpatient veterans age 50 and older (in 2003-04) in the VA, gender did not have any effect on vaccination for the 121,738 veterans surveyed[67]. Jha and coworkers evaluated multiple prevention and chronic disease measures in fiscal year 2000 and documented comparable overall care for both men and women overall in VA, although a few quality measures varied by age and sex[62]. Among those less than 65 years, women were more likely to receive hemoglobin A1c testing (OR 1.13, 95% CI 1.03-1.25) and adequate hypertension control (OR 1.09, 95% CI 1.00-1.18) but less likely to receive pneumococcal vaccine (OR 0.78, 95% CI 0.73-0.83). For patients age 65 and older, women were less likely to receive adequate hypertension control (OR 0.82, 95% CI 0.75-0.90) or pneumococcal vaccine (OR 0.92, 95% CI 0.86-0.99).

Tseng and colleagues performed 2 studies with veteran populations with diabetes. The first, which compared older male and female veterans with non-veterans enrolled in Medicare to examine gender differences in process of care measures, found no differences in glycosylated hemoglobin (HbA1c), or low density lipoprotein cholesterol (LDL-C) testing[59]. Women were more likely to have completed eye exams but less likely to have LDL-C under 130mg/dl compared with men.

In a separate diabetes study comparing female veterans with and without service connected disability status, women veterans with service connection were more likely to receive recommended diabetes tests compared with women veterans without service connection, but were less likely to have LDL-C controlled even though they were more likely to be tested[60]. The last study in this section focused on cardiovascular risks in veterans with HIV. Among HIV positive veterans started on protease inhibitors for disease control, 60% achieved the recommended lipid screening guidelines[63]. Notably, female gender was not a factor associated with receipt of lipid screening in either unadjusted or adjusted analyses.

The remaining three articles[64, 65, 68] described tobacco use and development of a tobacco cessation program for women veterans. Vander Weg[68] evaluated use of various tobacco products among the military by gender and noted use of any type of alternative tobacco products (e.g., bidics, cigars, kretekcs, pipes, and smokeless tobacco) was greater among cigarette smokers compared to non-cigarette smokers, and use of alternative products was consistently higher for males than for females. The qualitative articles described the development process for selecting ideal components of a smoking cessation program for women veterans and uncovered the finding that women veterans wanted both formal and informal support mechanisms (professional and peer support) in addition to *choice* for a smoking cessation program (new vs. traditional alcoholics anonymous style)[64]. When women in these focused groups were given a VA tailored smoking cessation booklet to choose options from, most women selected multiple options for cessation and least often chose the traditional VA program[65].

Surgical Outcomes

Four research studies focused on surgical outcomes in women patients or diseases predominant in women (e.g., breast cancer surgery)[69-72]. Johnson and colleagues evaluated post-operative morbidity and mortality among women patients (n=458 VA patients and n=3535 non-VA patients) undergoing vascular surgery at multiple VA and private hospitals[69]. In the stepwise logistic regression models adjusted for clinical and operative characteristics, VA and private sector hospitals showed no difference in mortality; however, VA care was associated with significantly lower morbidity (OR 0.60, 95% CI 0.44-0.81).

Fink and colleagues also evaluated post-operative morbidity and mortality among female surgical patients (n=5157 VA patients and n=27,467 non-VA patients) undergoing general surgery procedures in VA and private sector hospitals[71]. They found that risk adjusted morbidity was significantly lower in the VA compared with the private sector (OR 0.80, 95% CI 0.71-0.90), however, risk-adjusted mortality did not differ. The next study focused on surgical morbidity and mortality outcomes for breast surgery (n=1333) performed at VA hospitals over a 6-year period (1991-1997)[72]. Of those diagnosed with breast cancer (n=478), 75% were women. Thirty-day morbidity rates (12%), 30-day mortality rates (1%), and 1-year operation related readmission rates (<1%) were all low for both the women and men in VA. The most common post-operative complications were wound infections for both women and men, and urinary tract infections in women. Women breast cancer patients were more likely to be younger, unmarried, and low income compared with men.

The last study focused on surgical outcomes in VA and non-VA patients of both genders undergoing gastric bypass[70]. This surgical study evaluated 30-day post operative morbidity outcomes and predictors of morbidity in VA and non-VA male and female patients (veterans and non-veterans) undergoing Roux-en-Y gastric bypass surgery. The adjusted odds of post-operative morbidity for the VA versus non-VA female patients was 1.14 (95% CI 0.63-2.05), and for male patients was 2.29 (95%CI 1.28-4.10). Although the VA male subset showed high risk-adjusted postoperative morbidity, both the unadjusted or adjusted findings for VA females were equivalent to those of non-veteran females.

Prescribing Outcomes

We reviewed five studies that focused on prescribing outcomes[73-77]. In a VA and Medicare comparison paper, Barnett and colleagues found that VA users had lower rates of any inappropriate medication prescribed overall (21% vs. 29%, p<0.001), and the rate of inappropriate drug use was lower in VA compared with the private sector for males (21% vs. 24%, p<0.001) and females (28% vs. 32%, p<0.001)[75].

Three studies focusing only on VA populations showed that inappropriate prescribing was more likely to occur in VA women whether using Beers criteria[73], HEDIS 2006 criteria[74], or Zhan criteria[76]. In addition, gender-stratified analyses found that only geriatric care was protective against inappropriate prescribing for women. An additional study compared antidepressant treatment between the VA and private sector patients and found more than 80% of patients achieved guideline acute phase treatment (i.e., effective antidepressant medication therapy during the first 84 days after depression diagnosis) with little differences between VA and private sector[77]. Predictors of quality treatment included female gender, and comorbid substance abuse or other mental health diagnoses.

Pugh and colleagues identified inappropriate prescribing using multiple criteria (AHRQ, Beers, and Zhan)[76]. The Agency for Healthcare research and Quality (AHRQ) criteria included documentation of certain drugs by the categories of always avoid, rarely appropriate, or some indications while the Beers criteria involved the medications that should be avoided in persons aged 65 and older due to ineffectiveness or high risk to safety and medications that should not be used in older persons with specific conditions[99]. The AHRQ panel further identified situations in which use of rarely appropriate and some-indications drugs are proper (i.e., Zhan criteria). The study found that adjustment for clinical diagnoses decreased inappropriate prescribing practices from 33 to 23% of all veterans and showed that inappropriate drug exposure was prolonged (means not given). Multivariate analyses revealed that women were more likely than men to be prescribed inappropriate drugs using Zhan criteria (OR 1.3, 95% CI 1.2-1.3), and were less likely to receive dose-limited drugs (OR 0.6, 95% CI 0.6-0.7). Other factors associated with either inappropriate drugs or dose limited drugs were white race, psychiatric comorbidity, or receipt of an increasing number of medications.

Busch and colleagues, comparing the quality of pharmacotherapy for patients with major depression in the VA (n=27,713) and private sector (n=4852), found that over 80% of patients received guideline-level acute phase treatment (antidepressant therapy in first 84 days) in either system[77]. Raw scores showed that VA slightly outperformed the private sector with prescriptions for antidepressants in the initial 84 days (84.7% vs. 81.0%, p<.001) and maintenance phase treatment for 181 days (53.9% vs. 50.9%, p<.001). In the fully adjusted regression models, women patients were more likely to receive guideline level treatment at both 84 (OR 1.18, 95% CI 1.08-1.29) and 181 days (OR 1.14, 95% CI 1.07-1.22). The association of VA care with initial guideline treatment was lost after inclusion of co-morbid diagnoses. No difference was found between VA and private depression care quality in the fully adjusted model.

Cardiovascular Risk Reduction and Health Disparities

Nine studies possessed data on cardiovascular risk factors for women veterans, most in the form of prevalence of risk behaviors/conditions or comparisons of process and outcome measures as mentioned above[59, 60, 62, 63, 69, 70, 78-80]. Frayne et al assessed prevalence of known cardiac risk factors among women veterans who sustained a sexual assault while in the military, and identified obesity, smoking, hazardous alcohol use, sedentary lifestyle, and hysterectomy before age 40 as more common events in women reporting a history of sexual assault in the military compared with women without such as history[79]. Johnson et al identified watching television more than 2 hours per day and snacking/eating as significantly associated with obesity among women veterans after adjusting for patient characteristics and screening positive for depression or PTSD[78]. A study by Cypel and colleagues compared a national population based sample of female Vietnam veterans with non-Vietnam veteran cohorts, and found that women Vietnam veterans showed a significant deficit (ARR 0.78, 95% CI 0.62, 0.98) in circulatory system disease relative to non-Vietnam veterans, but significant deficits were also observed when both cohorts were compared with women in the U.S. population (SMR 0.65, 95% CI 0.54, 0.77; SMR 0.82, 95% CI 0.73, 0.93, respectively)[80]. Additionally, Vietnam veterans were at significantly greater risk of mortality from motor vehicle accidents than non-Vietnam veterans (ARR 2.60, 95% CI 1.22, 5.55) and this appeared to be specific to service in Vietnam based upon comparisons to the U.S. population. While each cardiovascular risk reduction and health disparities study evaluated cardiovascular risk factors or mortality in women veterans, none assessed risk reduction over time or due to specific therapy. The other six articles were mentioned in the sections on general quality of care prevention, processes and outcomes[59, 60, 62, 63] and surgical outcomes[69, 70].

Gender-specific and Reproductive Care

A range of articles of varying quality covered gender-specific and reproductive care issues[32, 41, 42, 81-91]. Three studies covered deployment related reproductive and pregnancy issues[32, 41, 42] and are discussed previously.

One narrative report[83] of a VA cognitive behavioral therapy program for transgender women veterans (male to female) showed improvement on measures of anxiety and depression from pre- to post-treatment and appeared to reduce transgender related isolation and stigma. Locating the group in the VA system felt supportive to the veterans who had conceptualized being rejected at a systemic level (e.g., by a government organization). Many transgender specific issues were addressed in this CBT framework, and the work may serve as a roadmap for future group and individual therapy.

Two studies involved urological issues in military or veteran patients[84, 87]. The first study reported that more active duty women with dysuria postponed voiding; reported fluid restriction; were treated for dysuria in the field or after field duty; and used tampons, pads or devices to control urinary incontinence during field duty[84]. The second study[87] described the prevalence of eight high priority urologic diseases among patients in the VA. While no major findings are reported by gender, interstitial cystitis was almost twice as prevalent among female compared to male VA users (2205 vs. 1311 per 100,000 persons). The etiology or context for this finding was not described.

One retrospective pilot study described pregnancy costs and outcomes at a single VA medical center [91]. These investigators found that among the 33 pregnancies reviewed, 31% were to women with at least one chronic condition (mainly hypertension and asthma), 39% had at least one psychiatric condition, and 36% had an adverse pregnancy outcome (e.g., premature birth, gestational diabetes, etc). The estimated mean total cost of pregnancy care for the entire sample was $9,359 (range $5,466 to $20,279).

A few studies provided information on sexual health, contraception and hormone therapy[81, 86, 88, 90]. Among a small group of active duty women completing an anonymous survey on sexual health information, responses yielded little desire for information regarding safer sexual practices[86]. However, information requested during normal duty differed from information requested for deployment. Information most frequently requested during deployment included how to abstain or say no to sex (23.5%), how to use safer sex or condoms (10.2%), and how to keep oneself clean or personal hygiene (9.2%), whereas no information (14.4%), how to use safer sex or condoms (9.3%), and how to abstain or say no to sex (9.3%) were the top choices for information requested during normal duty.

During 2004-2006, military facilities filled hormonal contraceptive prescriptions for more than half (54.2%) of all females who served in an active component of the US military[90]. The majority of females who were prescribed hormonal contraceptives were younger than 25 years old (51.2%), white (55%), and not married (56.7%). Females in their twenties were more likely than those younger or older to receive prescriptions for hormonal contraceptives of all types except the IUD with progestin. For latter reproductive years, two studies were present. In a very small study of women at one VA site, over three-quarters stopped taking hormone replacement therapy after the WHI trial reports in 2002, and recurrent vasomotor symptoms were common in those who quit abruptly compared to those who tapered[88]. Tapering did not appear to reduce the recurrence of vasomotor symptoms. A larger national study completed after the pilot, indicated similar findings with nearly two-thirds of women nationally in VA stopping their hormone therapy within two-years after the WHI trial[81].

Women with gender-specific and non-gender specific pain reported had high correlations with psychological stress, lower health status and sometimes trauma. For breast pain, women reporting frequent mastalgia, compared to those without mastalgia, were more likely to screen positive for PTSD, major depression, panic disorder, eating disorders, alcohol misuse, or domestic violence, and often reported fibromyalgia, chronic pelvic pain, or irritable bowel syndrome[89]. In a study of women veterans with and without menstrual symptoms, data revealed significantly lower scores for nearly all domains of the SF-36 ($p<.01$), both before and after adjustment for sociodemographic, psychosocial, and comorbidity variables[82]. Results remained unchanged when analyses were limited only to women without a depression or a sexual trauma history.

Finally, a mammogram intervention trial was evaluated for external and internal validity[85]. For internal validity, the five study groups did not differ with respect to any of the covariates. Groups not receiving the intervention showed similar rates of mammogram screening during the 1 or 2 years before or after the baseline survey, indicating that cueing had not occurred. Mammogram screening rates during the 30 months prior to the baseline evaluation for 5 different randomized groups of women showed mildly lower screening in group

5 compared to all other groups combined (82.3% vs 85.1%) which was consistent with changes occurring nationally. (The specific trial is discussed at the end of this quality section within the clinical trials subgroup.)

Other

Seven articles could not be clustered in the categories above[92-98]. One study focused on patient perceptions of breast cancer risk susceptibility and found that only breast symptoms and cancer worry predicted greater perceived susceptibility. The models only explained a small amount of variance for each susceptibility measure[98]. For VA patients on ace inhibitor medications, independent of other factors, risk of angioedema among VA patients was higher for blacks, females, and patients with chronic heart failure or coronary artery disease, but substantially lower for diabetics[92]. The five following studies had women in their samples and analyses and had no difference identified by gender[93, 95-97] and/or did not comment on results or discussions on implications of women in their sample for health status/quality of life comparisons[94, 95] or cost comparisons[93, 97].

Clinical Trials

The last two studies in this section are trials[8, 9]. One is an educational intervention to improve VA employee perceptions of women veterans. The other is an intervention to increase mammography screening among women veterans.

VA Employee Study

The VA employee study by Vogt[8] was an educational intervention which evaluated gender role ideology (i.e., "the extent to which a health-care worker does or does not rely on negative stereotypes about women, as they compare to men, to make judgments about different aspects of care"), knowledge, and sensitivity among male and female employees randomly given the educational training then compared with a control group[8]. Initial findings indicated that older age, direct patient contact, and years of VA employment predicted higher gender awareness and suggested a meaningful role for "hands-on" experience with veterans. Analyses revealed significantly greater improvement in sensitivity and knowledge for participants in intervention relative to control setting. Contrary to expectations, the program did not significantly improve gender-role ideology.

Mammography Intervention

This study by Vernon et al[9] was a randomized controlled trial of two interventions in a population-based, nationally representative sample of women veterans that compared rates of completion of two or more mammograms among women assigned to two types of interventions versus a survey only control group. While the absolute between group differences ranges from 3-6%, depending on analyses, neither was superior to the control group.

Summary

The satisfaction data are mixed. Women veterans who do not use the VA lack understanding of VA care and services. Among VA users, women and men had similar outpatient satisfaction ratings; however, women had consistently lower ratings for inpatient care. Additionally, women veteran satisfaction was affected by access to women's clinics, gynecological care, and overall continuity of care. The VA quality assessment indicated that women in VA may have some comparable outcomes with men; however, overall improvement is needed for lipid and hypertension control and preventive immunizations. Surgical data indicate that women in VA settings have equal or lower surgical morbidity and mortality outcomes compared with the private sector for general and vascular procedures. Pharmacy data indicate that while VA has consistently lower or comparable rates of inappropriate prescription drugs in the elderly, and women in the VA (compared to men) are consistently more likely to be prescribed inappropriate drugs by regardless of the criteria used[73-76].

Separately, the literature on quality of care and cardiovascular risks in women veterans is salient but small. Women appear to have obesity related surgical outcomes equivalent or better than the non-veteran women, but have higher levels of cardiovascular disorders compared to civilian women and lower level of ambulatory care intermediate outcomes (LDL-cholesterol control) compared to men veterans. None of the epidemiologic or quality of care studies focused on cardiac risk reduction over time or with specific therapies. Studies with intermediate outcomes (e.g., controlled lipids or other process measures) and disease outcomes (lower disease-specific morbidity and mortality rates) are desperately needed to understand what improves cardiovascular care for women veterans alone or in mixed populations with men.

Finally, women veterans with a history of MST and PTSD have increased obesity associated risk factors. This subgroup of studies indicates that cardiovascular risk reduction will be a growing and ongoing need in VA with the growing population of women veterans who will age in our system.

ACCESS AND UTILIZATION

Forty-eight articles focused on access and utilization addressed determinants of access, gender and utilization, and utilization among special populations – sexual trauma patients, mental health/PTSD patients, and veterans from different periods of military service. Twelve articles focused on determinants of access[51, 100-110]; fourteen focused on gender-specific care or gender differences and access[46, 81, 111-122]. Six articles focused on sexual trauma patients and utilization[123-128]; and eleven focused on PTSD or other mental health patients and utilization[15, 129-138]. Five additional studies focused on access and utilization among specific cohorts of veterans[20, 25, 139-141].

General Determinants of Access

The studies on determinants of access to VA care identified knowledge gaps about VA care, incorrect assumptions about services available to women, and difficulty with using VA care as major barriers to women's using the VA[51, 101, 102]. Other factors influencing women not to use the VA or to use both the VA and private sector care included availability of private insurance or higher income[102-104]. Patient and organizational factors related to low VA and non-VA dual use were no insurance, receipt of general gynecological care from the VA provider or use of women's clinics[100, 107]. For patients older than 65, availability of Medicare HMOs predicted healthcare use outside the VA[110]. Among veterans with dual VA-Medicare eligibility, veteran women were more likely than veteran men to rely solely on VA care[108, 109]. Additionally, one qualitative study found that veterans reported using VA due to cost issues in addition to more access to services (compared to local community) and quality of care available at VA[106]. These veterans voiced similar concerns about cost, access and quality in other settings if VA outsourced care, with the greatest concerns being whether they would be negative effects (e.g., lower quality, harder to obtain appointments or wait time)[106]. One last study on utilization after increases in medication copayments among male and female veterans with schizophrenia noted that outpatient visits remained stable, but inpatient admissions increased slightly[105].

Gender-Specific Differences in Access

Compared with male VA users, women who used VA care had more outpatient encounters[111] and also used more outpatient services if they had medical, mental health, or pain conditions in comparison to men[111, 112, 115]. Women veterans in a Midwestern regional sample were found to have higher health related quality of life compared with men; however, younger women who had poor mental or physical health functioning had fewer primary care visits compared with men with the same characteristics[114]. A study of total knee replacement or hip arthroplasty in the VA found no gender difference in rates of these surgical procedures[117]. A smoking cessation study documented that while women and men were equally likely to be advised to quit smoking and be referred to a cessation program, women less often received nicotine patches (OR 0.50, 95% CI 0.3, 0.9) and were less likely to have successfully quit smoking one year later[118]. For women veterans requiring emergency gynecological or mental health care, VA sites reported high availability during general clinic hours (64.4% and 82.7% respectively had specialty emergency care); however, this access dropped to half or fewer sites offering after hours emergency care for women[46]. The main predictors for access for a VA site were the presence of a separate women's health clinic or lower local managed care penetration for emergency mental health.

Gender-Specific Differences in Utilization

The gender-specific data covered a broad range of topics. After the Women's Health Initiative data were reported in 2002 and 2004, women veterans nationally discontinued hormone therapy at about the same rate as non-veteran women. However women utilizing VA women's clinics more often stayed on hormone therapy compared with women cared for in other VA settings[81]. Women veterans with spinal cord disorders compared with those without showed higher rates of cardiovascular disease, lower health status, and fewer reports of preventive dental care, colon screening, and mammogram screening, indicating areas for improvement. Rates of vaccinations and lipid screening were similar for these two groups[113]. With regard to breast disease, image-guided breast biopsies were shown to be more cost-effective compared with traditional open biopsy surgical techniques at one VA site[116], and factors inversely affecting demand for mammograms included patient characteristics of older age, poor health and smoking status, and the system factor of increased waiting time for the mammogram[119].

LaVcla[122] also described utilization of services by veterans with spinal cord disorders. Females, older, and non-white veterans (p<.0.000 each), and veterans with a history of medical problems such as respiratory, kidney/urinary tract, circulatory, or digestive system diseases (p<0.005 for each) were more likely to use outpatient care, and farther distance from VA facilities indicated infrequent use (p<0.000). Homeless female veterans were more likely to receive compensation benefits rather than pension benefits[120]. In the limited number of veterans (15%) who were subsequently awarded benefits; they were more likely to have reported recent use of VA services and a greater number of medical and psychiatric problems at the time of outreach[120]. Finally, a convenience sample of women veterans at one VA site[121] showed that women veterans with pain (vs. without) were more than 6 times as likely to report ≥12 medical visits in the past year and twice as likely to report ≥12 visits to a mental health provider.

Sexual Trauma and Utilization

The research on sexual trauma and utilization revealed patient difficulties with identifying their emotions[124], more use of VA services among those with sexual trauma histories[125, 128], and more psychological impairment compared with veterans with other forms of trauma[126, 128]. In addition, women who had experienced more severe forms of sexual violence in the military (i.e., repeated rapes or gang rapes) were severely impaired physically and emotionally compared with women who had no or one such event, and were more likely to use both inpatient and outpatient mental health services[127]. A national study of veterans screened for military sexual trauma showed that both men and women who had a positive screen were more than twice as likely to have a post-screen mental health visit compared with those who screened negative[123], a benefit for both genders in the VA.

PTSD and Other Mental Health Issues

Among the eleven PTSD and mental health studies focused on utilization[15, 129-138], women with PTSD symptoms and women with other mental health issues were more likely to use VA services compared with women without PTSD symptoms or men, respectively[129, 138]. Other gender-related findings were that being mistreated as a child did not appear to be associated with increased utilization among women with PTSD[133]. Both women veterans with PTSD and female partners of Vietnam Veterans with PTSD preferred treatment or support services that were female-only[135, 136]. One study examined continuity of care and treatment outcomes but was not able to find a significant association between continuity of care factors and PTSD outcomes when analyses were adjusted for multiple comparisons[137]. Compared to men with mental illness, women with mental health issues were less likely to be placed in nursing home settings[132]. Identification of patients by psychiatric criteria on interview indicated that up to 44% of women veterans in primary care may have at least 1 mental health diagnosis[130], and middle age adults are more likely to have a psychiatric diagnosis compared with younger and older veterans[131]. One article noted that patients with mental health diagnoses (compared to those without mental illness) are less likely to be screened for lipid disorders unless they have increased outpatient utilization at the VA[134]. A last study focusing on OEF/OIF veterans with PTSD is discussed in a previous section[15].

Access and Utilization Among Specific Cohorts

Several access and utilization studies focused on specific cohorts of military personnel. One study noted that active duty Air Force personnel who self-refer for mental health services compared with those referred by supervisors are less likely to have a significant diagnosis, have confidentiality broken, or have career-affecting recommendations made[140]. For women Vietnam veterans, physical health problems mediated the relationship between combat exposure and outpatient utilization for physical health, whereas combat exposure only indirectly predicted men's mental healthcare use [139]. The Iowa Gulf War Study identified similar combat and noncombat exposures among men and women but noted that women were more likely to report more than 5 outpatient visits in the prior year, and inpatient hospitalization, and receive VA compensation[141]. Two other studies focused on OEF/OIF personnel and were discussed previously[20, 25].

Summary

Women with positive screens for mental health disorders, trauma, or diagnoses tend to use more healthcare services than women without positive screens or than men veterans. In a few areas, findings are mixed, cautioning us to remain aware of patients who may reduce utilization because of specific mental health issues.

PSYCHIATRIC CONDITIONS

The 85 publications covering mental health and psychiatric issues fell into five broad categories: PTSD[5-7, 13, 15, 22, 23, 26, 28, 55, 58, 129, 131, 133, 135-137, 142-166]; substance abuse and treatment[167-171]; general mental health[130, 132, 134, 138, 140, 172-179]; Trauma[10, 124, 128, 180-194]; and other[77, 105, 195-199]. The PTSD focused articles included screening and treatment, descriptors and determinants of diagnosis, quality of life and utilization impacts, and comorbid disorders. General mental health articles included prevention and screening, deployment issues, quality of life, and utilization.

PTSD

Clinical Trials

Three PTSD clinical trials focused on treatment occurred during this period[5-7]. David evaluated a 12-week open behavioral intervention for PTSD patients[5]. The intervention focused on structured group psychotherapy and self-defense training and measured patient risk perceptions among women veterans with PTSD. Women veterans showed significant and sustained improvement at both 3 and 6 months after completing the program with respect to PTSD avoidance behavior and hyperarousal symptoms. Patients also had decreased depression scores, and increased interpersonal self-efficacy, self defense self-efficacy and willingness to participate in community activities. Schnurr et al. was a multi-site trial that randomized women veterans and female military personnel with PTSD to either prolonged exposure therapy or present-centered therapy by standard protocol for 10 weeks[6]. This study indicated that prolonged exposure therapy was significantly associated with a greater reduction of PTSD symptoms and a lower likelihood of meeting PTSD diagnostic criteria after therapy was completed. A final pilot trial by Butterfield et al. evaluated olanzapine therapy over 10 weeks in a small, double blind, placebo controlled group of patients (predominantly female) with noncombat related PTSD and reported no between-group difference in treatment responses but noted a large placebo effect[7].

Screening and Symptoms

PTSD screening and treatment included seven articles covering a variety of topics[26, 28, 135, 137, 142-144]. One study found that a small subset of veterans (2.7%) filing disability benefits for PTSD reported being spontaneously distressed by a survey[142]. However, in a Persian Gulf War I cohort, gender analyses revealed that perceived threat was associated with more PTSD type symptoms for National Guard/Reserve men compared with active duty men, but the PTSD symptom associations were greater for active duty women compared with women in guard/reserve units[143]. Another gender related finding was that the most important factor for women veterans and partners of disabled veterans coming to the VA for PTSD treatment was the availability of specialized treatment programs for women[135].

Women veterans treated for PTSD with group psychoeducation and self-defense training showed (similar to the David 2006 study[5]) improved use of personal safety skills[144]. Lambert's case series on the use of aripiprazole with either sertraline or cognitive –behavior therapy shows some promise in improving symptoms in some patients[26]. Corrections for multiple comparisons eliminated the relationships between clinical status outcomes and continuity of care in a small sample of women receiving outpatient VA treatment for PTSD[137]. Future clinical trials will be needed to produce clinical evidence for improving PTSD symptoms in women through medication and therapy.

Finally, the findings of the repeat post-deployment screens for PTSD and other symptoms among OEF/OIF veterans are discussed in an earlier section[28].

Determinants of Diagnosis

Twelve articles focused on determinants of a diagnosis[22, 23, 133, 145-153]. In a study of stress and social support among male and female Marine recruits, the negative impact of stress reactions on hardiness (i.e., courage and motivation to cope with stressors in daily life) was strongest when social support was low; however, in women stress reactions predicted enhanced hardiness when social support was high[145]. Women who have strong social supports may endure more stressors without negative consequences. In a similar fashion, life experiences and unit cohesion predicted PTSD symptoms in active duty soldiers, with unit cohesion appearing to ameliorate some life experiences and symptoms[153]. A few studies focused on the determinants of PTSD found the following associations: 1) poorer perceptions of health and well being were correlated with increased depression or PTSD symptoms[146]; 2) PTSD diagnosis and symptoms were associated with more medical conditions and poorer health related quality of life[151], and gender did not moderate the relationship between PTSD and poorer health related quality of life[147]; 3) one VA primary care clinic identified PTSD as the best predictor for somatization in women patients[148]; and 4) pain related factors[149], childhood non-sexual/physical maltreatment, childhood sexual assault[152] or adult sexual assault[133, 150] were significant predictors of PTSD symptom clusters among women veterans. Two other studies are discussed previously in the deployment and post-deployment health section[22, 23].

Quality of Life and PTSD

Fifteen articles focused on quality of life and mental health[13, 15, 55, 58, 129, 131, 136, 154-161]. Findings varied in mixed gender versus single gender studies. Among male and female veterans treated for PTSD in the VA, overall quality of life was poor and did not differ between genders, and numbing was uniquely associated with reduced quality of life[154]. In contrast, women screening positive for PTSD symptoms (compared to those screening negative) had more mental and physical problems, and poorer health related quality of life[160].

Two studies examined how PTSD-related stress affects the family of veterans[155, 156]. Severity of PTSD symptoms was negatively correlated with marital adjustment (r=-.38), family adaptability (r=-.40), cohesion (r=-.34) and parenting satisfaction (r=-.31)[155]. Among women Vietnam veterans, hyperarousal symptoms negatively impacted parenting satisfaction[156]. Gahm et al. identified family experiences that may contribute to PTSD risk[161]. Experiencing combat (OR 2.04), witnessing someone being assaulted or killed (OR 1.88), and number of adverse childhood events (OR 1.25) all emerged as significant risk factors for PTSD symptoms[161]. In a PTSD disability benefits study, regional differences in PTSD awards are not explained by different PTSD symptom severity or level of disability[159]. Separately, no difference in the reporting of low income occurs among women compared to men applying for PTSD disability benefits[157]. In addition, a disparity in estimated rates of service connection for PTSD by gender was partially explained by differences in combat exposure[158]. A number of related articles were discussed under postdeployment OEF/OIF health[13, 15] and PTSD symptoms related to access and utilization[129, 131, 136].

Satisfaction had mixed associations with PTSD symptoms[55, 58]. Women veterans with trauma related mental health symptoms reported more satisfaction with overall primary care and their provider[55]. However, in another study patients with PTSD and other co-morbid diagnoses reported lower overall satisfaction with primary care (see Desai (2005) discussion under quality of care and patient satisfaction)[58].

Comorbid Disorders

A few articles covered co-morbid disorders[162-166]. Women with PTSD had more medical conditions and worse health status than women with only depression or neither diagnosis[162]. Among a male and female cohort of Persian Gulf military followed longitudinally, a drug problem or PTSD symptoms at time point 2 was predictive of a positive drug use screen at time point 3 but not predictive of alcohol use[163]. African American female veterans at one VA site had a greater prevalence of prior exposure to violence (childhood or adult sexual abuse, intimate partner violence or sexual harassment) than their Caucasian counterparts, but these levels were not markedly different from other low-income African American women[164]. In another single site VA study of women veterans, women with a history of MST had a greater odds of PTSD (OR 4.4, 95% CI 2.4, 8.2), but prior experience of other trauma was not a significant predictor of PTSD (OR 1.3, 95% CI 0.63, 2.5)[165]. A similar analysis revealed that the relative risk of women with MST developing PTSD was nearly 2.5 times that of patients without MST (RR 2.40)[166].

Substance Abuse and Treatment

Five studies explored substance abuse issues in military and veteran populations[167-171]. Two[169, 170] describe military and veteran characteristics associated with alcohol use, while the others describe predictors for participating in substance abuse treatment programs[167, 168, 171].

Gutierrez and researchers[169] assessed alcohol behaviors among deployed soldiers (within and outside of the United States) in 2003 and found that significant predictors of greater alcohol-related consequences, as assessed with the CAGE questionnaire, included less formal education, male gender, not being in an intimate relationship, racial/ethnic minority status, enlisted rank, having been deployed to the continental United States, and greater stress [$\chi^2(8,5,458) = 235.991; p < 0.001$]. Lande et al[170] determined gender based differences in alcohol use among Army soldiers and noted that although men were more likely to engage in "bolus" (binge) drinking, women exceeded established guidelines for safe alcohol consumption (i.e., 7 drinks per week) at a risk-adjusted rate nearly twice that of men. In addition, for individuals whose behaviors were considered unsafe, the severity of reported negative consequences was influenced by gender. Women initially experience greater psychosocial impairment, and—should harmful drinking patterns progress to alcohol dependency – they are at greater risk of injury, morbidity, and mortality than men.

Predictors of admission into a substance abuse treatment program for active duty women include coexisting psychiatric conditions[171], primarily concurrent use of alcohol[171] and for veteran women in intensive outpatient treatment include cocaine abuse/dependence, greater burden of medical and psychiatric co-morbidities compared to men in intensive treatment and compared to other women veterans not in treatment[167]. For homeless veterans, the situation is more complicated. Benda[168] compared readmission rates for substance abuse program by gender among homeless veterans and identified abuse in childhood, during military status or in the recent 2 year period prior to admission were all potent factors for women compared to men. Readmission for women was heightened by increases in depression, suicidal thoughts or traumatic events, while for men it was increased by elevated substance abuse, aggression and cognitive impairment. However, social supports through family, friends, church or other mechanism all lessened readmission rates for women, while employment stability and job satisfaction reduced the readmissions for men.

General Mental Health

The general mental health prevention and screening articles indicated that women in the military had a higher prevalence of mental health disorders such as panic, anxiety and depression compared with men in the military[175, 176]. The exception is alcohol abuse, where the prevalence among men in active duty cohorts was higher than that of military women[175].

Quality of Life

For veterans responding to the Large Health Survey of Veteran Enrollees in 1999, Physical and mental component scores were similar by gender except among those age 65 or older, where mean MCS was better for women than men (49.3 vs 45.9, p<.001)[179]. Among women veterans, health related quality of life physical component scores were lower, with more limitations in activities of daily living and more reported pain than the men[172], and among psychiatric patients, rural veterans had worse physical component scores and mental component scores compared to urban-dwelling veterans[173]. Those with mental health comorbidities also had lower health related quality of life scores[174]. Women in the Air Force showed increased levels of family stress, work family conflicts and job distress compared with community samples of women[177], and children of deployed Air Force mothers in Operation Desert Storm were at risk for multiple behavioral and emotional adjustments problems[178].

Utilization

Within VA primary care clinics, a large proportion of women (44%) had at least one mental health diagnosis, and about 40% of these women with a mental health condition received care in a VA specialized mental health clinic[130]. Service members discharged from the military for mental health reasons were more likely to use VA mental health services if they were women, older, or had schizophrenia or bipolar disorder. The women were more likely to contact VA and use VA services compared with the men[138]. Within the military, service members who self-referred for mental health care had better outcomes than those members who had been referred to mental health care by their supervisor[140]. Other articles discussed previously included nursing home users were likely to be men, recently hospitalized and with dementia[132], and lipid screening was low for veterans who used VA mental health services infrequently but increased screening occurred with increased levels of outpatient use[134].

Trauma

General Sexual Trauma or MST

Key findings from the nine articles on general sexual trauma or MST[10, 124, 128, 180-185] include the following: Positive MST screens among women and men were associated with greater odds of nearly all mental health comorbidities, including PTSD in women (OR 8.83, 99% CI 8.34, 9.35) and men (OR 3.00, 99% CI 2.89, 3.12), but were almost three times stronger among women[180]. These findings were reinforced in an additional study evaluating the various forms of sexual assault and PTSD diagnosis[183] and in one of the OEF/OIF deployment studies discussed previously[10]. In-service sexual harassment severity was also associated with PTSD symptom severity in women, after adjusting for other reported traumas[185]. Many active duty women (80%) and men (45%) reported at least one type of sexual stressor in the previous year (i.e., sexual identity challenges, sexual harassment, or sexual assault)[181]. In addition, women with a history of sexual trauma report significantly higher levels of anxiety for any gender-specific or invasive exams (breast, pelvic, rectal) when the clinician is male (p<.001 for each exam)[182]. Moreover, women with sexual trauma histories showed evidence of alexithymia (i.e., difficulty identifying one's emotions), and this factor explained variance in both physical health and urgent care utilization among these women[124]. Notably, a small study of women with physical and/or sexual assault histories reported that self-defense training would be an effective addition to traditional treatments for PTSD[184]. An additional relevant article is discussed in the access and utilization section[128].

Trauma from Multiple Sources

Women experiencing multiple traumatic events (sexual, physical or both) during military service, had more severely impacted health status[190, 194] and more outpatient visits[190]. Some women had repeated violent experiences from childhood which were also associated with worse physical and mental quality of life compared to women without the history[189]; other childhood events were more frequently perpetrated by parental figures, occurred over longer durations or involved more severe experiences of abuse[186]. Prior to entering the military, one-fourth of recruits reported pre-military physical intimate partner violence (IPV) events[191] and both physical IPV and history of interpersonal trauma predicted attrition from the military[187, 191]. Separately, active duty women's perceptions of screening for domestic violence (now called intimate partner violence) in the military was generally supportive, but fewer women thought abuse should be reported to the commanding officer[192].

Multiple workplace factors increased the likelihood of physical assault for women in the military: experiencing unwanted sexual advances or pressure for dates in sleeping quarters (7 fold); experiencing hostile work environments (5 fold); observing heterosexual activities in sleeping quarters (4 fold); and ranking officers making sexually demeaning comments or behaviors (3 fold)[193]. Of note, being quartered in mixed gender barracks was not significantly associated with physical assault. Combat and non-combat exposed veterans had different levels of sexual assault in-service; higher levels occurred among non-combat males (13% vs 6%) and non-combat females (75% vs 63%) for unclear reasons[188].

Other

The other mental health articles focused on other psychiatric conditions not discussed previously. Three articles focused on depression treatment[77, 197, 199]. The first showed no difference in depression therapy between VA and the private sector[77], the second identified depression screening rates of nearly 85% in 2002, but only about half the patients received follow up if they screened positive and male gender was a factor[197]. The third article found that among depressed veterans, being young, male, and white were the demographic factors associated with higher suicide risks[199]. However, the relative risk ratio for suicide among men compared with women was smaller than in the general population. The remaining four articles identified that 60% of veterans with serious mental illness had overwhelmingly poor dental health[195]; bipolar disorder patients who were nonadherent to medication were likely to have an active substance use disorder such as alcohol abuse[196], with women showing higher odds of nonadherence[198]; and lastly, psychiatric drug refills dropped nearly 25% among schizophrenia patients after copayments for medications increased[105].

The remaining articles from on psychiatric conditions were included in the access and utilization section covering mental health issues, deployment and post-deployment health section for OEF/OIF veterans and non OEF/OIF veterans.

Summary

The section on psychiatric conditions covers a broad spectrum of literature describing issues for women and men veterans. This literature should provide a stable foundation for increasing treatment and outcome pilot and multi-center trial studies among women veterans. Three points should be emphasized.

- More clinical trials like those of David, Schnurr, and Butterfield are needed to help direct VA providers toward treatment options that are best suited for the female veteran patient.
- The literature confirms the positive relationship between MST and PTSD, and both of these diagnoses have multiple negative health-related associations that both providers and policymakers need to understand. In particular, women with a sexual trauma history reported significant anxiety for any invasive exam and male providers. Such data are critical for managing patients in primary care where repeated invasive exams (breast, pelvic, rectal) will be required to provide evidence-based quality care over the life span; the role of provider type and practice setting (women's clinics) may be a long-term issue.
- A small cluster of studies show that social support (in military or in civilian life) may be a factor for resiliency and quality of life among women and (possibly their children) while performing in the military and when they transition home from deployment.

SUMMARY AND DISCUSSION

The growth in the number of women in the military is reshaping the veteran population, with women now constituting one of the fastest growing segments of eligible VA healthcare users. This trend has been accelerated by the unexpectedly high VA enrollment of women veterans from recent wars in Iraq and Afghanistan. As women veterans have entered the VA healthcare system in increasing numbers, VA managers and providers have been challenged to organize and deliver gender-specific and gender-sensitive services in a system that has otherwise historically focused on treating men. Gender-specific care also imposes considerable training and experience requirements on a VA workforce with limited exposure to female patients.

VA's health services research enterprise has been designed to map to high priority topics, women veterans' health and health care among them. Yano and colleagues led the leadership efforts for the first mapping of VA research priorities to the needs of women veterans with the VA Women's Health Research Agenda Setting Conference in late 2004[200]. This initial women's health research agenda was the product of a national consensus development meeting, which (a) brought together researchers from various fields (laboratory, clinical science, rehabilitation and health services) to focus on establishing an evidence base for a women's health agenda and (b) to incorporate results of the first VA systematic review of the literature on women veterans[1]. That review identified 182 relevant articles published between 1978 and 2004. Most were descriptive in nature, using observational study designs; only 2 were randomized controlled trials. About 45% of the studies were VA funded, with the majority of the literature focusing on women veterans' mental health (mostly risk, prevalence and treatment of PTSD) and general health services research (8 on quality of care, 5 on patient satisfaction, 25 on use and organization of care).

In the current updated systematic review, we identified 195 articles from 2004-2008–more articles in 5 years than we identified in the previous 25 years. This sharp increase in volume is likely due to VA's increased focus on research funding in these priority areas. Consistent with the previous systematic review, most VA women's health research continues to be observational; however, more articles are shifting from a descriptive to an analytical focus (i.e., determinants of care or health), and there were 5 clinical trials, a modest increase from the first review.

While the focus on mental health among women in the military and women veterans remains high, with a continuing emphasis on PTSD and MST, important new work has been published on prevalence of mental health conditions in different settings and for different subgroups and on non-trauma-related mental health problems (e.g., depression, serious mental illness). Emphasis on access, utilization and quality of care for women veterans has also increased, with a rapidly emerging focus on post-deployment health. These topic areas clearly map to ongoing VA research priorities, demonstrated in part by the fact that about 60% of the articles were VA funded in whole or in part, up from 45% in the review published in 2006.

BUILDING KNOWLEDGE: NOTABLE RESEARCH ADVANCES

To what extent has the more recent literature closed the gaps identified in the previous review? Previous notable gaps included very limited information on the prevalence of chronic diseases, women veterans' preferences and self-reported care needs, research on utilization patterns within and outside the VA health care system, transitions from military to veteran status, studies of the quality of care women veterans receive, and studies on how to improve their quality of care. These gaps served as the basis for more targeted solicitations for new research.

We highlight 3 areas with the noteworthy impact:

1) Treatment outcomes in PTSD: The Schnurr study is the first multi-centered, VA funded cooperative trial focused on outcomes of women veterans with PTSD using a comparison of prolonged exposure therapy to a previous standard of care. Due to the quality of the research and significant clinical findings, prolonged exposure therapy is being considered by VA administration as part of the revised guidelines for PTSD standards of care due out later this year, used to train clinical providers, and implemented across the field nationally[6].

2) Access to care: We now know more about barriers, perceptions and utilization of VA care among women veterans, and this information should be used as a foundation to remove barriers and consider methods for restructuring care to meet healthcare needs. Chief barriers include knowledge gaps and incorrect assumptions about VA services among women veterans outside the VA and high use of care once enrolled in VA among women with various co-morbidities. This knowledge should direct us toward potential interventions among subgroups of women veterans to decrease barriers and documented and improved care outcomes among women in VA with significant co-morbidities.

3) Organizational determinants of quality care: Advances in research describing how care is organized for women in VA demonstrate variations in service availability and their determinants as well as the importance of practice environment for women veterans care. Better attention to gynecologic access (staff, clinic, services) appears to be important for types of services a woman has access to and a key area for future research in VA. The impact of local leadership on women veteran services also appears essential. Future

quality improvement interventions need to consider the integration of leadership or other diverse stakeholders in care of women.

Separately, the PTSD trial impacts the literature on women veterans in another manner. Few studies had an adequate sample for comparing women to men or VA users to non-users and evaluating outcomes. The Schnurr trial overcame this challenge and future studies should use similar methods (multi-site approach, cooperative study, practice based research network) to achieve adequate patient samples for clinical and health services research Schnurr trial[6]. The Schnurr trial tackles the historical research dilemma of insufficient sampling strategies for performing primary or subgroup analyses of women in VA and demonstrates that it is feasible to conduct robust clinical trials in women veterans[201].

With the current systematic review, we found increases in the number of articles on access, utilization and quality of care studies. Collectively, this research provides an evidence base for detecting barriers to VA care that women soldiers may encounter, defining optimal women's healthcare delivery arrangements, and adopting best practices. In these areas, the field as a whole is now ready to move toward identifying and implementing interventions to promote best practices. This identification of interventions and promotion of best practices fits within the VA Quality Enhancement Research Initiative (QUERI) model for translational research and quality improvement[202]. The VA QUERI program promotes the linking of research and clinical practice to improve the quality and outcomes of care among veterans across the VA system by a series of quality improvement steps and interventions that involve researchers, providers, and clinical managers[203]. These steps include: (1) identifying high-risk or high burden conditions or problems; (2) identify best practices or clinical guidelines; (3)define variations from best practices and their determinants; (4) identify and implement interventions to promote best practices; (5) assess intervention program feasibility, outcomes and impacts on patient, provider, and system; and (6) assess intervention program impacts on health releated quality of life outcomes[203, 204]. VA women veterans' health research now stands solidly within the VA QUERI framework at steps 3 and 4, where variations can be identified and explicitly understood so that appropriate interventions will be designed for women veterans.

ONGOING GAPS: FUTURE VA RESEARCH TARGETS

In contrast to the growth in the scientific literature on access, utilization and quality, recently funded VA studies have not yet made their mark in the published literature on prevalence of chronic diseases or on transitions from military to veteran status. Additional areas that stand as new or ongoing gaps in the literature for our women veteran population are included below:

1) Limited clinical and intervention outcome data for chronic physical or mental health conditions and complex combinations of diseases
2) Limited information on transitions from military to civilian life
3) Minimal information of military duty and transitions on families
4) Health issues for women veterans across the life span (e.g., pregnancy, aging)
5) New information on general care or gender differences for veterans with polytrauma or traumatic brain injury
6) Challenges and strategies for comanaging mental health and general preventive health

We anticipate that the increases in VA women's health services research funding over the past 5 years will continue to affect the topical coverage and methodological diversity and rigor seen in the coming 5 years. Ongoing efforts to continually update the literature, augmented by interactive search capabilities, will enhance the value and application of this growing evidence base to ongoing care improvements in health care settings within and outside the VA. Separately, we suggest that internal final reports of VA supported research should document if the study contained findings reportable by gender (whether the same or different) even if that was not *one* of the research aims of the study. Such detailing offers insight to unknown areas of disparity or equity in veteran health and healthcare.

The primary limitation of this systematic review, as with any review, is the potential for having missed salient articles. Search terms for our topic area of women veterans' health and health care have not been standardized in such as way that authors routinely select consistent terms. We thus augmented traditional computerized search strategies with contacts among leading researchers in the field in the hopes of enhancing our yield. Now that we have a significant database of relevant articles, we hope that authors not represented herein will forward their articles for inclusion. As with any systematic review, we are also limited by publication bias.

CONCLUSIONS

The areas more fully developed in women veterans' research (access, utilization, and quality of care) will serve as a foundation for future intervention and implementation research in VA. In addition, the already substantial scope of women veteran mental health literature should be expanded with future VA studies on treatment modalities and outcomes and should explore ways in which veteran, provider, or practice settings can incorporate potential treatments.

FUTURE RESEARCH

Continued need exists for clinical trials data involving women veteran health issues and women veteran populations.

REFERENCES

1.   Goldzweig, C. L., et al., The State of Women Veterans' Health Research. Journal of General Internal Medicine, 2006. 21: p. S82-S92.

2.   Hayes, P. and M. Krauthamer, Changing the face of health care for women veterans. Federal Practitioner, 2009. 26(2): p. 8-10.

3.   Brix, K., RE: Women Veteran Literature Request, B. Bean-Mayberry, Editor. 2008: Los Angeles.

4.   Jadad, A. R., et al., Assessing the quality of reports of randomized clinical trials: is blinding necessary? Control Clin Trials, 1996. 17(1): p. 1-12.

5.   David, W. S., T. L. Simpson and A. J. Cotton, Taking charge: a pilot curriculum of self-defense and personal safety training for female veterans with PTSD because of military sexual trauma. J Interpers Violence, 2006. 21(4): p. 555-65.

6.   Schnurr, P. S., et al., Cognitive Behavioral Therapy for Posttraumatic Stress Disorder in Women. JAMA, 2007. 297.

7.   Butterfield, M. I., et al., Olanzapine in the treatment of post-traumatic stress disorder: a pilot study. International Clinical Psychopharmacology, 2001. 16(4): p. 197-203.

8.   Vogt, D. S., A. A. Barry and L. A. King, Toward Gender-Aware Health Care: Evaluation of an Intervention to Enhance Care for Female Patients in the VA Setting. Journal of Health Psychology, 2008. 13(5): p. 624-638.

9.   Vernon, S. W., et al., Promoting regular mammography screening II: Results from a randomized controlled trial in US women veterans. J Natl Cancer Inst, 2008. 100: p. 347-358.

10. Smith, T. C., et al., Prior assault and posttraumatic stress disorder after combat deployment. Epidemiology, 2008. 19: p. 505-512.

11. Felker, B., et al., Characteristics of deployed Operation Iraqi Freedom military personnel who seek mental health care. Mil Med, 2008. 173(2): p. 155-8.

12. Seal, K. H., et al., Bringing the war back home: mental health disorders among 103,788 US veterans returning from Iraq and Afghanistan seen at Department of Veterans Affairs facilities. Arch Intern Med, 2007. 167(5): p. 476-82.

13. Hoge, C. W., et al., Association of posttraumatic stress disorder with somatic symptoms, health care visits, and absenteeism among Iraq war veterans. Am J Psychiatry, 2007. 164(1): p. 150-3.

14. Helmer, D. A., et al., Health and exposure concerns of veterans deployed to Iraq and Afghanistan. J Occup Environ Med, 2007. 49(5): p. 475-80.

15.   Erbes, C., et al., Post-traumatic stress disorder and service utilization in a sample of service members from Iraq and Afghanistan. Mil Med, 2007. 172(4): p. 359-63.

16.   Katz, L. S., et al., Women who served in Iraq seeking mental health services: Relationships between military sexual trauma, symptoms, and readjustment. Psychological Services, 2007. 4(4): p. 239-249.

17.   Hoge, C. W., et al., Combat duty in Iraq and Afghanistan, mental health problems, and barriers to care. N Engl J Med, 2004. 351(1): p. 13-22.

18.   Stetz, M. C., et al., Psychiatric diagnoses as a cause of medical evacuation. Aviat Space Environ Med, 2005. 76(7 Suppl): p. C15-20.

19.   Rundell, J. R., Demographics of and diagnoses in Operation Enduring Freedom and Operation Iraqi Freedom personnel who were psychiatrically evacuated from the theater of operations. Gen Hosp Psychiatry, 2006. 28(4): p. 352-6.

20.   Hoge, C. W., J. L. Auchterlonie and C. S. Milliken, Mental health problems, use of mental health services, and attrition from military service after returning from deployment to Iraq or Afghanistan. JAMA, 2006. 295(9): p. 1023-32.

21.   Mental health encounters and diagnoses following deployment to Iraq and/or Afghanistan, US Armed Forces, 2001-2006. Medical Surveillance Monthly Report, 2007. 14(4): p. 2-8.

22.   Lapierre, C. B., A. F. Schwegler and B. J. Labauve, Posttraumatic stress and depression symptoms in soldiers returning from combat operations in Iraq and Afghanistan. J Trauma Stress, 2007. 20(6): p. 933-43.

23.   Smith, T. C., et al., New onset and persistent symptoms of post-traumatic stress disorder self reported after deployment and combat exposures: prospective population based US military cohort study. BMJ, 2008. 336(7640): p. 366-71.

24.   Seal, K. H., et al., Getting beyond "Don't ask; don't tell": an evaluation of US Veterans Administration postdeployment mental health screening of veterans returning from Iraq and Afghanistan. Am J Public Health, 2008. 98(4): p. 714-20.

25.   McNulty, P. A., Reported stressors and health care needs of active duty Navy personnel during three phases of deployment in support of the war in Iraq. Mil Med, 2005. 170(6): p. 530-5.

26.   Lambert, M. T., Aripiprazole in the management of post-traumatic stress disorder symptoms in returning Global War on Terrorism veterans. Int Clin Psychopharmacol, 2006. 21(3): p. 185-7.

27.   Stecker, T., et al., An assessment of beliefs about mental health care among veterans who served in Iraq. Psychiatr Serv, 2007. 58(10): p. 1358-61.

28. Routine screening and referrals for Post-Traumatic Stress Disorder (PTSD) after returning from Operation Iraqi Freedom in 2005, US Armed Forces. Medical Surveillance Monthly Report, 2007. 14(6): p. 2-7.

29. Farley, J. H., et al., Far forward gynecologic care of the female soldier. J Reprod Med, 2006. 51(1): p. 31-5.

30. Thomson, B. A. and P. E. Nielsen, Women's health care in Operation Iraqi Freedom: a survey of camps with echelon I or II facilities. Mil Med, 2006. 171(3): p. 216-9.

31. Vogt, D. S., Validation of Scales From the Deployment Risk and Resilience Inventory in a Sample of Operation Iraqi Freedom Veterans. Assessment, 2008. 15(4): p. 391-403.

32. Haas, D. M. and L. A. Pazdernik, Partner deployment and stress in pregnant women. J Reprod Med, 2007. 52(10): p. 901-6.

33. Adler, A. B., et al., The impact of deployment length and experience on the well-being of male and female soldiers. J Occup Health Psychol, 2005. 10: p. 121-37.

34. Vogt, D. S., et al., Deployment Stressors, Gender, and Mental Health Outcomes Among Gulf War I Veterans. Journal of Traumatic Stress, 2005. 18(3): p. 272-284.

35. Lindstrom, K. E., et al., The mental health of U.S. military women in combat support occupations. J Womens Health (Larchmt), 2006. 15(2): p. 162-72.

36. Cavin, S., World War II Never Ended in My House: Interviews of 12 Office of Strategic Services Veterans of Wartime Espionage on the 50th Anniversary of WW II, in *Psychobiology of posttraumatic stress disorders: A decade of progress (Vol. 1071)*. 2006, Blackwell Publishing, 2006, xxiii, 547 Blackwell Publishing: Malden, MA Malden, MA. p. 463-471.

37. Wolfe, J., P. J. Brown and M. L. Bucsela, Symptom responses of female Vietnam veterans to Operation Desert Storm. Am J Psychiatry, 1992. 149(5): p. 676-9.

38. Smith, T. C., et al., The physical and mental health of a large military cohort: baseline functional health status of the Millennium Cohort. Bmc Public Health, 2007. 7.

39. Pierce, P. F., Physical and emotional health of Gulf War veteran women. Aviat Space Environ Med, 1997. 68(4): p. 317-21.

40. Smith, T. C., et al., The occupational role of women in military service: validation of occupation and prevalence of exposures in the Millennium Cohort Study. Int J Environ Health Res, 2007. 17(4): p. 271-84.

41. Araneta, M. R., et al., Conception and pregnancy during the Persian Gulf War: the risk to women veterans. Ann Epidemiol, 2004. 14(2): p. 109-16.

42. Pierce, P. F., C. Antonakos and B. A. Deroba, Health care utilization and satisfaction concerning gender-specific health problems among military women. Mil Mcd, 1999. 164(2): p. 98-102.

43.   Bean-Mayberry, B. A., et al., Organizational characteristics associated with the availability of women's health clinics for primary care in the Veterans Health Administration. Military Medicine, 2007. 172(8): p. 824-8.

44.   Seelig, M. D., et al., Availability of gynecologic services in the Department of Veterans Affairs. Womens Health Issues, 2008. 18(3): p. 167-73.

45.   Bean-Mayberry, B. A., et al., Federally Funded Comprehensive Women's Health Centers: Leading Innovation in Women's Healthcare Delivery. Journal of Women's Health, 2007. 16(9): p. 1281-1290.

46.   Washington, D. L., et al., VA emergency health care for women: condition--critical or stable? Womens Health Issues, 2006. 16(3): p. 133-8.

47.   Cope, J. R., et al., Determinants of contraceptive availability at medical facilities in the Department of Veterans Affairs. J Gen Intern Med, 2006. 21 Suppl 3: p. S33-9.

48.   Hall, M. E., et al., Military sexual trauma services for women veterans in the Veterans Health Administration: The patient-care practice environment and perceived organizational support. Psychological Services, 2007. 4(4): p. 229-238.

49.   Yano, E. M., et al., Diffusion of Innovation in Women's Health Care Delivery: The Department of Veterans Affairs' Adoption of Women's Health Clinics. Women's Health Issues, 2006. 16: p. 226-235.

50.   Bean-Mayberry, B., C. C. Chang and S. H. Scholle, Brief Report: Lack of a Race Effect in Primary Care Ratings among Women Veterans. Journal of General Internal Medicine, 2006. 21(10): p. 1105-1108.

51.   Washington, D. L., et al., Women Veterans' Perceptions and Decision-Making about VA Health Care. Military Medicine, 2007.

52.   Bean-Mayberry, B. A., et al., Patient Satisfaction in Women's Clinics Versus Traditional Primary Care Clinics in the Veterans Administration. Journal of General Internal Medicine, 2003. 18: p. 175-181.

53.   Wright, S. M., et al., Patient satisfaction of female and male users of Veterans Health Administration services. J Gen Intern Med, 2006. 21 Suppl 3: p. S26-32.

54.   Bean-Mayberry, B. A., et al., Ensuring high-quality primary care for women: predictors of success. Womens Health Issues, 2006. 16(1): p. 22-9.

55.   Lang, A. J., et al., Mental health and satisfaction with primary health care in female patients. Womens Health Issues, 2005. 15(2): p. 73-9.

56.   Harriott, E. M., T. V. Williams and M. R. Peterson, Childbearing in U.S. military hospitals: dimensions of care affecting women's perceptions of quality and satisfaction. Birth, 2005. 32(1): p. 4-10.

57.   Fan, V. S., et al., Continuity of care and other determinants of patient satisfaction with primary care. J Gen Intern Med, 2005. 20(3): p. 226-33.

58.   Desai, R. A., E. A. Stefanovics and R. A. Rosenheck, The role of psychiatric diagnosis in satisfaction with primary care: data from the department of veterans affairs. Med Care, 2005. 43(12): p. 1208-16.

59.   Tseng, C. L., et al., Are there gender differences in diabetes care among veterans? Journal of General Internal Medicine 2006. 21(S3): p. S47-53.

60.   Tseng, C. L., et al., Diabetes care among veteran women with disability. Womens Health Issues, 2006. 16(6): p. 361-71.

61.   Etzioni, D. A., et al., Measuring the quality of colorectal cancer screening: the importance of follow-up. Dis Colon Rectum, 2006. 49(7): p. 1002-10.

62.   Jha, A. K., et al., Quality of ambulatory care for women and men in the Veterans Affairs Health Care System. J Gen Intern Med, 2005. 20(8): p. 762-5.

63.   Korthuis, P. T., et al., Lipid screening in HIV-infected veterans. J Acquir Immune Defic Syndr, 2004. 35(3): p. 253-60.

64.   Katzburg, J. R., et al., Listen to the consumer: designing a tailored smoking-cessation program for women. Substance Use & Misuse, 2008. 43(8-9): p. 1240-1259.

65.   Katzburg, J. R., et al., Combining Women's Preferences & Expert Advice to Design a Tailored Smoking Cessation Program. Subst Use Misuse, 2009. 44(14): p. 2114-37.

66.   Friedemann-Sanchez, G., J. M. Griffin and M. R. Partin, Gender differences in colorectal cancer screening barriers and information needs. Health Expect, 2007. 10(2): p. 148-60.

67.   Straits-Troster, K. A., et al., Racial/ethnic differences in influenza vaccination in the Veterans Affairs Healthcare System. Am J Prev Med, 2006. 31(5): p. 375-82.

68.   Vander Weg, M., et al., Prevalence of alternative forms of tobacco use in a population of young adult military recruits. Addictive Behaviors, 2008. 33(1): p. 69-82.

69.   Johnson, R. G., et al., Comparison of Risk-Adjusted 30-Day Postoperative Mortality and Morbidity in Department of Veterans Affairs Hospitals and Selected University Medical Centers: Vascular Surgical Operations in Women. Journal of American College of Surgeons, 2007. 204: p. 1137-1146.

70.   Lautz, D. B., et al., Bariatric operations in Veterans Affairs and selected university medical centers: results of the patient safety in surgery study. J Am Coll Surg, 2007. 204(6): p. 1261-72.

71.   Fink, A. S., et al., Comparison of risk-adjusted 30-day postoperative mortality and morbidity in Department of Veterans Affairs hospitals and selected university medical centers: general surgical operations in women. J Am Coll Surg, 2007. 204(6): p. 1127-36.

72.   Hynes, D. M., et al., Breast cancer surgery trends and outcomes: results from a National Department of Veterans Affairs study. J Am Coll Surg, 2004. 198(5): p. 707-16.

73.   Bierman, A. S., et al., Sex differences in inappropriate prescribing among elderly veterans. Am J Geriatr Pharmacother, 2007. 5(2): p. 147-61.

74.   Pugh, M. J., et al., Assessing potentially inappropriate prescribing in the elderly Veterans Affairs population using the HEDIS 2006 quality measure. J Manag Care Pharm, 2006. 12(7): p. 537-45.

75.   Barnett, M. J., et al., Comparison of rates of potentially inappropriate medication use according to the Zhan criteria for VA versus private sector medicare HMOs. J Manag Care Pharm, 2006. 12(5): p. 362-70.

76.   Pugh, M. J., et al., Potentially inappropriate prescribing in elderly veterans: are we using the wrong drug, wrong dose, or wrong duration? J Am Geriatr Soc, 2005. 53(8): p. 1282-9.

77.   Busch, S. H., D. L. Leslie and R. A. Rosenheck, Comparing the quality of antidepressant pharmacotherapy in the Department of Veterans Affairs and the private sector. Psychiatr Serv, 2004. 55(12): p. 1386-91.

78.   Johnson, K. M., K. M. Nelson and K. A. Bradley, Television Viewing Practices and Obesity Among Women Veterans. Journal of General Internal Medicine, 2006. 21: p. S76-81.

79.   Frayne, S., et al., Sexual assault while in the military: Violence as a predictor of cardiac risk? Violence & Victims, 2003. 18(2): p. 219-225.

80.   Cypel, Y. and H. Kang, Mortality patterns among women Vietnam-era veterans: Results of a retrospective cohort study. Annals of Epidemiology, 2008. 18(3): p. 244-252.

81.   Haskell, S. G., et al., Determinants of Hormone Therapy Discontinuation among Female Veterans Nationally. Military Medicine, 2008. 173(1): p. 91-6.

82.   Barnard, K., et al., Health status among women veterans with menstrual symptoms. Journal of Women's Health 2003. 12(9): p. 911-920.

83.   Maguen, S., J. C. Shipherd and H. N. Harris, Providing Culturally Sensitive Care for Transgender Patients. Cognitive and Behavioral Practice, 2005. 12: p. 479-490.

84.   Albright, T. S., et al., Acute Dysuria among Female Soldiers. Military Medicine, 2005. 170(9): p. 735-738.

85.   del Junco, D. J., et al., Promoting regular mammography screening I. A systematic assessment of validity in a randomized trial. J Natl Cancer Inst, 2008. 100(5): p. 333-46.

86.   von Sadovszky, V. and N. Ryan-Wenger, Army women's sexual health information needs. J Obstet Gynecol Neonatal Nurs, 2007. 36(4): p. 348-57.

87.   Sohn, M. W., et al., Prevalence and trends of selected urologic conditions for VA healthcare users. BMC Urol, 2006. 6: p. 30.

88.   Haskell, S. G., After the Women's Health Initiative: Postmenopausal women's experiences with discontinuing estrogen replacement therapy. J Womens Health (Larchmt), 2004. 13(4): p. 438-42.

89.   Johnson, K. M., et al., Frequency of mastalgia among women veterans: Association with psychiatric conditions and unexplained pain syndromes. Journal of General Internal Medicine Improving health care for women veterans., 2006. 21(Suppl 3): p. S70-S75.

90.   Hormonal contraceptive use among female service members, active components, U.S. Armed Forces, January 2004-March 2006. Medical Surveillance Monthly Report, 2007. 14(7): p. 9-13.

91.   Chireau, M. V., et al., Outcomes, costs, and utilization of pregnancy related care. Federal Practitioner, 2006: p. 20-30.

92.   Miller, D. R., et al., Angioedema incidence in US veterans initiating angiotensin-converting enzyme inhibitors. Hypertension, 2008. 51(6): p. 1624-30.

93.   Yu, W., T. H. Wagner and P. G. Barnett, Determinants of cost among people who died in VA nursing homes. Med Care Res Rev, 2006. 63(4): p. 477-98.

94.   Weeks, W. B., et al., Rural-urban disparities in health-related quality of life within disease categories of Veterans. J Rural Health, 2006. 22(3): p. 204-11.

95.   Mrus, J. M., et al., Health-related quality of life in veterans and nonveterans with HIV/AIDS. J Gen Intern Med, 2006. 21 Suppl 5: p. S39-47.

96.   McEachrane-Gross, F. P., J. M. Liebschutz and D. Berlowitz, Use of selected complementary and alternative medicine (CAM) treatments in veterans with cancer or chronic pain: a cross-sectional survey. BMC Complement Altern Med, 2006. 6: p. 34.

97.   Maciejewski, M. L., et al., The performance of administrative and self-reported measures for risk adjustment of Veterans Affairs expenditures. Health Serv Res, 2005. 40(3): p. 887-904.

98.   McQueen, A., et al., Predictors of perceived susceptibility of breast cancer and changes over time: a mixed modeling approach. Health Psychol, 2008. 27(1): p. 68-77.

99.   Fick, D. M., et al., Updating the Beers criteria for potentially inappropriate medication use in older adults: results of a US consensus panel of experts. Arch Intern Med, 2003. 163(22): p. 2716-24.

100.   Bean-Mayberry, B., et al., Comprehensive Care for Women Veterans: Indicators of Dual Use of VA and non-VA Providers. Journal of American Medical Women's Association, 2004. 59(3): p. 192-197.

101.   Vogt, D. S., et al., Barriers to Veterans Health Administration Care in a Nationally Representative Sample of Women Veterans. Journal of General Internal Medicine, 2006. 21: p. S19-S25.

102. Washington, D. L., et al., To Use or Not to Use: What Influences Why Women Veterans Choose VA Health Care. Journal of General Internal Medicine, 2006. 21: p. S11-S18.

103. Shen, Y., et al., The impact of private insurance coverage on veterans' use of VA care: insurance and selection effects. Health Serv Res, 2008. 43(1 Pt 1): p. 267-86.

104. Ross, J. S., et al., Dual use of Veterans Affairs services and use of recommended ambulatory care. Med Care, 2008. 46(3): p. 309-16.

105. Zeber, J. E., et al., Effect of a medication copayment increase in veterans with schizophrenia. Am J Manag Care, 2007. 13(6 Pt 2): p. 335-46.

106. Wakefield, B. J., et al., Veterans' use of Department of Veterans Affairs care and perceptions of outsourcing inpatient care. Mil Med, 2007. 172(6): p. 565-71.

107. Nelson, K. M., G. A. Starkebaum and G. E. Reiber, Veterans using and uninsured veterans not using Veterans Affairs (VA) health care. Public Health Rep, 2007. 122(1): p. 93-100.

108. Mooney, S. E. and W. B. Weeks, Where do women veterans get their inpatient care? Womens Health Issues, 2007. 17(6): p. 367-73.

109. Hynes, D. M., et al., Veterans' access to and use of Medicare and Veterans Affairs health care. Med Care, 2007. 45(3): p. 214-23.

110. Shen, Y., et al., VA-Medicare dual beneficiaries' enrollment in Medicare HMOs: access to VA, availability of HMOs, and favorable selection. Med Care Res Rev, 2005. 62(4): p. 479-95.

111. Frayne, S. M., et al., Gender and Use of Care: Planning for Tomorrow's Veterans Health Administration. Journal of Women's Health, 2006. 16(8): p. 1188-1199.

112. Frayne, S. M., et al., Gender Disparities in Veterans Health Administration Care: Importance of Accounting for Veteran Status. Medical Care, 2008. 46(5): p. 549-553.

113. LaVela, S., et al., Disease Prevalence and Use of Preventive Services: Comparison of Female Veterans in General and Those with Spinal Cord Injuries and Disorders. MS. Journal of Women's Health, 2006.

114. Singh, J. A. and M. Murdoch, Effect of Health Related Quality of Life on Women and Men's Veterans Affairs (VA) Health Care Utilization and Mortality. Journal of General Internal Medicine, 2007. 22(9): p. 1260-1267.

115. Kaur, S., et al., Gender differences in health care utilization among veterans with chronic pain. J Gen Intern Med, 2007. 22(2): p. 228-33.

116. Hatmaker, A. R., et al., Cost-effective use of breast biopsy techniques in a Veterans health care system. Am J Surg, 2006. 192(5): p. e37-41.

117. Borrero, S., et al., Brief report: Gender and total knee/hip arthroplasty utilization rate in the VA system. J Gen Intern Med, 2006. 21 Suppl 3: p. S54-7.

118.   Sherman, S. E., et al., Gender differences in smoking cessation services received among veterans. Womens Health Issues, 2005. 15(3): p. 126-33.

119.   Lairson, D. R., W. Chan and G. R. Newmark, Determinants of the demand for breast cancer screening among women veterans in the United States. Soc Sci Med, 2005. 61(7): p. 1608-17.

120.   Chen, J. H., et al., Receipt of disability through an outreach program for homeless veterans. Mil Med, 2007. 172(5): p. 461-5.

121.   Haskell, S. G., et al., The prevalence and age-related characteristics of pain in a sample of women veterans receiving primary care. J Womens Health (Larchmt), 2006. 15(7): p. 862-9.

122.   LaVela, S. L., et al., Geographical proximity and health care utilization in veterans with SCI&D in the USA. Soc Sci Med, 2004. 59(11): p. 2387-99.

123.   Kimerling, R., et al., Evaluation of Universal Screening for Military-Related Sexual Trauma. Psychiatric Services, 2008. 59: p. 635-640.

124.   Polusny, M. A., et al., The Role of Cumulative Sexual Trauma and Difficulties Identifying Feelings in Understanding Female Veterans' Physical Health Outcomes. Gen Hosp Psychiatry, 2008. 30(2): p. 162-70.

125.   Kelly, M. M., et al., Effects of Military Trauma Exposure on Women Veterans' Use and Perceptions of Veteran Health Administration Care. Journal of General Internal Medicine, 2008. 23(6): p. 741-747.

126.   Zinzow, H. M., et al., Sexual assault, mental health, and service use among male and female veterans seen in Veterans Affairs primary care clinics: a multi-site study. Psychiatry Res, 2008. 159(1-2): p. 226-36.

127.   Sadler, A. G., B. M. Booth and B. N. Doebbeling, Gang and multiple rapes during military service: health consequences and health care. J Am Med Womens Assoc, 2005. 60(1): p. 33-41.

128.   Stein, M. B., et al., Relationship of sexual assault history to somatic symptoms and health anxiety in women. Gen Hosp Psychiatry, 2004. 26(3): p. 178-83.

129.   Dobie, D. J., et al., PTSD Screening Status is Associated with Increased VA Medical and Surgical Utilization in Women. Journal of General Internal Medicine, 2006. 21: p. S58-64.

130.   Grubaugh, A., et al., Female Veterans Seeking Medical Care at Veterans Affairs Primary Care Clinics: Psychiatric and Medical Illness Burden and Service Use. Women & Health, 2006. 43(3): p. 41-62.

131.   Frueh, B. C., et al., Age differences in posttraumatic stress disorder, psychiatric disorders, and healthcare service use among veterans in Veterans Affairs primary care clinics. Am J Geriatr Psychiatry, 2007. 15(8): p. 660-72.

132. Miller, E. A. and R. A. Rosenheck, Risk of nursing home admission in association with mental illness nationally in the Department of Veterans Affairs. Med Care, 2006. 44(4): p. 343-51.

133. Lang, A. J., et al., Relationships among childhood maltreatment, PTSD, and health in female veterans in primary care. Child Abuse Negl, 2006. 30(11): p. 1281-92.

134. Kaplowitz, R. A., et al., Health care utilization and receipt of cholesterol testing by veterans with and those without mental illness. Gen Hosp Psychiatry, 2006. 28(2): p. 137-44.

135. Fontana, A. and R. Rosenheck, Treatment of female veterans with posttraumatic stress disorder: the role of comfort in a predominantly male environment. Psychiatr Q, 2006. 77(1): p. 55-67.

136. Sherman, M. D., et al., Mental health needs of cohabiting partners of Vietnam veterans with combat-related PTSD. Psychiatr Serv, 2005. 56(9): p. 1150-2.

137. Greenberg, G. A., A. Fontana and R. A. Rosenheck, Continuity and intensity of care among women receiving outpatient care for PTSD. Psychiatr Q, 2004. 75(2): p. 165-81.

138. Mojtabai, R., et al., Use of VA aftercare following military discharge among patients with serious mental disorders. Psychiatric Services, 2003. 54(3): p. 383-388.

139. Maguen, S., et al., Predictors of mental and physical health service utilization among Vietnam veterans. Psychological Services, 2007. 4(3): p. 168-180.

140. Rowan, A. B. and R. L. Campise, A multisite study of Air Force outpatient behavioral health treatment-seeking patterns and career impact. Mil Med, 2006. 171(11): p. 1123-7.

141. Carney, C. P., et al., Women in the Gulf War: combat experience, exposures, and subsequent health care use. Mil Med, 2003. 168(8): p. 654-61.

142. Halek, K., M. Murdoch and L. Fortier, Spontaneous Reports of Emotional Upset and Health Care Utilization Among Veterans With Posttraumatic Stress Disorder After Receiving a Potentially Upsetting Survey. American Journal of Orthopsychiatry, 2005. 75(1): p. 142-151.

143. Vogt, D. S., et al., Deployment Stressors and Posttraumatic Stress Symptomatology: Comparing Active Duty and National Guard/Reserve Personnel from Gulf War I. Journal of Traumatic Stress, 2008. 21(1): p. 66-74.

144. Westrup, D. A., J. C. Weitlauf and J. Keller, I Got My Life Back! Making a Case for Self Defense Training for Older Women with PTSD. Clinical Gerontologist Vol 28(3) (2005):, 2005. 28(3): p. 113-118.

145. Vogt, D. S., et al., Longitudinal Investigation of Reciprocal Relationship Between Stress Reactions and Hardiness. Personality and Social Psychology Bulletin, 2008. 34(1): p. 61-73.

146.   Mancino, M. J., et al., Quality-adjusted health status in veterans with posttraumatic stress disorder. J Nerv Ment Dis, 2006. 194(11): p. 877-9.

147.   Ouimette, P., et al., Posttraumatic stress disorder and health status among female and male medical patients. J Trauma Stress, 2004. 17(1): p. 1-9.

148.   Escalona, R., et al., PTSD and somatization in women treated at a VA primary care clinic. Psychosomatics, 2004. 45(4): p. 291-6.

149.   Asmundson, G. J., K. D. Wright and M. B. Stein, Pain and PTSD symptoms in female veterans. Eur J Pain, 2004. 8(4): p. 345-50.

150.   Lang, A. J., et al., Direct and indirect links between childhood maltreatment, posttraumatic stress disorder, and women's health. Behavioral Medicine, 2008. 33(4): p. 125-135.

151.   Monnier, J., et al., US female veterans in VA primary care: post traumatic stress disorder symptoms and functional status. Primary Care Psychiatry, 2004. 9(4): p. 145-150.

152.   Becker, M., The impact of childhood adversity factors on posttraumatic stress and other functioning in adult women veterans. Dissertation Abstracts International Section A: Humanities and Social Sciences, 2006. 66(8-A): p. 2830.

153.   Brailey, K., et al., PTSD symptoms, life events, and unit cohesion in U.S. soldiers: baseline findings from the neurocognition deployment health study. J Trauma Stress, 2007. 20(4): p. 495-503.

154.   Schnurr, P. S. and C. A. Lunney, Exploration of how gender differences in quality of life relates to posttraumatic stress disorder in male and female veterans. Journal of Rehabilitation Research and Development, 2008. 45(3): p. 383-394.

155.   Gold, J. I., et al., PTSD Symptom Severity and Family Adjustment Among Female Vietnam Veterans. Military Psychology, 2007. 19: p. 72-81.

156.   Berz, J. B., et al., Associations Between PTSD Symptoms and Parenting Satisfaction in a Female Veteran Sample. Journal of Psychological Trauma, 2008. 7(1): p. 37-45.

157.   Murdoch, M., et al., Mitigating Effect of Department of Veterans Affairs Disability Benefits for Post-Traumatic Stress Disorder on Low Income. Military Medicine, 2005. 170(2): p. 137-140.

158.   Murdoch, M., et al., Gender Differences in Service Connection for PTSD. Medical Care, 2003. 41(8): p. 950-961.

159.   Murdoch, M., et al., Regional variation and other correlates of Department of Veterans Affairs Disability Awards for patients with posttraumatic stress disorder. Med Care, 2005. 43(2): p. 112-21.

160.   Dobie, D. J., et al., Posttraumatic stress disorder in female veterans: association with self-reported health problems and functional impairment. Arch Intern Med, 2004. 164(4): p. 394-400.

161. Gahm, G. A., et al., Relative impact of adverse events and screened symptoms of post-traumatic stress disorder and depression among active duty soldiers seeking mental health care. Journal of Clinical Psychology, 2007. 63(3): p. 199-211.

162. Frayne, S. M., et al., The burden of medical illness in women with depression and PTSD. Archives of Internal Medicine 2004. 164(12): p. 1306-1312.

163. Shipherd, J. C., J. Stafford and L. R. Tanner, Predicting alcohol and drug abuse in Persian Gulf War veterans: What role do PTSD symptoms play? Addictive Behaviors, 2005. 30: p. 595-599.

164. Campbell, R., et al., The co-occurrence of childhood sexual abuse, adult sexual assault, intimate partner violence, and sexual harassment: A mediational model of posttraumatic stress disorder and physical health outcomes. Journal of Consulting and Clinical Psychology, 2008. 76(2): p. 194-207.

165. Yaeger, D., et al., DSM-IV diagnosed posttraumatic stress disorder in women veterans with and without military sexual trauma. Journal of General Internal Medicine, 2006. 21: p. S65-S69.

166. Himmelfarb, N., D. Yaeger and J. Mintz, Posttraumatic stress disorder in female veterans with military and civilian sexual trauma. Journal of Traumatic Stress, 2006. 19(6): p. 837-846.

167. Stecker, T., et al., Characteristics of women seeking intensive outpatient substance use treatment in the VA. J Womens Health (Larchmt), 2007. 16(10): p. 1478-84.

168. Benda, B., A Study of Substance Abuse, Traumata, and Social Support Systems Among Homeless Veterans. Journal of Human Behavior in the Social Environment Vol 12(1) (2005): 59-82, 2005. 12(q): p. 59-82.

169. Gutierrez, C. A., et al., Predictors of aversive alcohol consequences in a military sample. Mil Med, 2006. 171(9): p. 870-4.

170. Lande, R. G., et al., Gender differences and alcohol use in the US Army. J Am Osteopath Assoc, 2007. 107(9): p. 401-7.

171. Dove, M. B. and H. J. Joseph, Sociodemographic profile of women entering a military substance use disorder treatment center. Mil Med, 2007. 172(3): p. 283-7.

172. Teh, C. F., et al., Gender differences in health-related quality of life for veterans with serious mental illness. Psychiatr Serv, 2008. 59(6): p. 663-9.

173. Wallace, A. E., et al., Rural and urban disparities in health-related quality of life among veterans with psychiatric disorders. Psychiatr Serv, 2006. 57(6): p. 851-6.

174. Forman-Hoffman, V. L., et al., Mental health comorbidity patterns and impact on quality of life among veterans serving during the first Gulf War. Quality of Life Research, 2005. 14(10): p. 2303-2314.

175. Riddle, J. R., et al., Millennium Cohort: the 2001-2003 baseline prevalence of mental disorders in the U.S. military. J Clin Epidemiol, 2007. 60(2): p. 192-201.

176. Gahm, G. A. and B. A. Lucenko, Screening soldiers in outpatient care for mental health concerns. Mil Med, 2008. 173(1): p. 17-24.

177. Vinokur, A., P. Pierce and C. Buck, Work-family conflicts of women in the Air Force: their influence on mental health and functioning. J Organizational Behav, 1999. 20: p. 865-878.

178. Pierce, P., A. Vinokur and C. Buck, Effects of war-induced maternal separation on children's adjustment during the Gulf War and two years later. J Appl Soc Psychol, 1998. 14: p. 1287-1312.

179. Frayne, S. M., et al., Health status among 28,000 women veterans: The VA Women's Health Program Evaluation Project. Journal of General Internal Medicine 2006. 21(S3): p. S40-46.

180. Kimerling, R., et al., The Veterans Health Administration and Military Sexual Trauma. American Journal of Public Health, 2007. 97: p. 2160-2166.

181. Murdoch, M., et al., Functioning and Psychiatric Symptoms among Military Men and Women Exposed to Sexual Stressors. Military Medicine, 2007. 172(7): p. 718-725.

182. Lee, T. T., et al., Impact of clinician gender on examination anxiety among female veterans with sexual trauma: a pilot study. J Womens Health (Larchmt), 2007. 16(9): p. 1291-9.

183. Suris, A., et al., Sexual assault in women veterans: an examination of PTSD risk, health care utilization, and cost of care. Psychosom Med, 2004. 66(5): p. 749-56.

184. David, W. S., et al., Making a case for personal safety: perceptions of vulnerability and desire for self-defense training among female veterans. J Interpers Violence, 2004. 19(9): p. 991-1001.

185. Murdoch, M., et al., The Association between In-service Sexual Harassment and Post-traumatic Stress Disorder among Department of Veterans Affairs Disability Applicants. Military Medicine, 2006. 171(2): p. 166-73.

186. Schultz, J. R., et al., Child Sexual Abuse and Adulthood Sexual Assault among Military Veteran and Civilian Women. Military Medicine, 2006. 171(8): p. 723-728.

187. Wolfe, J., et al., Gender and Trauma as Predictors of Military Attrition: A Study of Marine Corps Recruits. Military Medicine, 2005. 170(12): p. 1037-1043.

188. Murdoch, M., et al., Prevalence of In-Service and Post-Service Sexual Assault among Combat and Noncombat Veterans Applying for Department of Veterans Affairs Posttraumatic Stress Disorder Disability Benefits. Military Medicine, 2004. 169(5): p. 392-395.

189. Suris, A., et al., Mental health, quality of life, and health functioning in women veterans: differential outcomes associated with military and civilian sexual assault. J Interpers Violence, 2007. 22(2): p. 179-97.

190. Sadler, A. G., et al., Life span and repeated violence against women during military service: effects on health status and outpatient utilization. J Womens Health (Larchmt), 2004. 13(7): p. 799-811.

191. Merrill, L. L., et al., Premilitary intimate partner violence and attrition from the U.S. Navy. Mil Med, 2006. 171(12): p. 1206-10.

192. Gielen, A. C., et al., Domestic violence in the military: women's policy preferences and beliefs concerning routine screening and mandatory reporting. Mil Med, 2006. 171(8): p. 729-35.

193. Sadler, A. G., et al., The military environment: risk factors for women's non-fatal assaults. J Occup Environ Med, 2001. 43(4): p. 325-34.

194. Sadler, A. G., et al., Health-related consequences of physical and sexual violence: women in the military. Obstet Gynecol, 2000. 96(3): p. 473-80.

195. Kilbourne, A. M., et al., Oral health in Veterans Affairs patients diagnosed with serious mental illness. J Public Health Dent, 2007. 67(1): p. 42-8.

196. Sajatovic, M., et al., Self-reported medication treatment adherence among veterans with bipolar disorder. Psychiatr Serv, 2006. 57(1): p. 56-62.

197. Desai, M. M., R. A. Rosenheck and T. J. Craig, Case-finding for depression among medical outpatients in the veterans health administration. Medical Care, 2006. 44(2): p. 175-181.

198. Copeland, L. A., et al., Treatment adherence and illness insight in veterans with bipolar disorder. Journal of Nervous and Mental Disease, 2008. 196(1): p. 16-21.

199. Zivin, K., et al., Suicide mortality among individuals receiving treatment for depression in the Veterans Affairs health system: associations with patient and treatment setting characteristics. Am J Public Health, 2007. 97(12): p. 2193-8.

200. Yano, E. M., et al., Toward a VA women's health research agenda: Setting evidence-based priorities to improve the health and health care of women veterans J Gen Intern Med, 2006. 21(S3): p. S93-S101.

201. Yano, E. M., et al., Integration of women veterans into VA quality improvement research efforts: what researchers need to know. J Gen Intern Med, 2010. 25 Suppl 1: p. 56-61.

202. McQueen, L., B. S. Mittman and J. G. Demakis, Overview of the Veterans Health Administration (VHA) Quality Enhancement Research Initiative (QUERI). J Am Med Inform Assoc, 2004. 11(5): p. 339-43.

203. Rubenstein, L. V., et al., From understanding health care provider behavior to improving health care: the QUERI framework for quality improvement. Quality Enhancement Research Initiative. Med Care, 2000. 38(6 Suppl 1): p. I129-41.

204. Yano, E. M., The role of organizational research in implementing evidence-based practice: QUERI Series. Implement Sci, 2008. 3: p. 29.

APPENDIX 1. SCREENER FORM

Article ID:
Reviewer:
Date:
Author:
Title:

1. Inclusion/Exclusion Criteria: (CHECK YES/NO)

   A. Study relates to US veterans or military
   Personnel.................................... ☐ YES ☐ NO→STOP

   B. Study includes women veterans, compares men and
   women, or analyzes women
   separately .... ☐ YES ☐ NO

   C. Study involves active duty military and involves a
   health condition or functional status that requires
   medical intervention.............. ☐ YES ☐ NO

   D. Topic is relevant to VA healthcare or how VA care is
   delivered to women .... ☐ YES ☐ NO

   IF NO FOR B,C, AND D →STOP

2. Design:

   Study Type: (CIRCLE ONE ONLY)

   Descriptive study
   (has no hypothesis or statistical testing) 1

   Observational study
   (assesses the effect of an intervention,
   risk or prognosis, knowledge, attitudes,
   or beliefs, etc.)...2

   Experimental studies 3

   Qualitative research 4

   Systematic review or Meta-analysis 5

   Non-systematic review .... 6 →STOP

   Editorial/ commentary .... 7 →STOP

   Unclear.. 8 →STOP

   Data Source/Sampling: (ANSWER AS APPLICABLE)

   Sample size:_____ ☐non-patient

   Total sample size(if men):_____

   Setting:

   Clinic☐ Hospital☐ Int. HCS☐ Multi-site☐
   City☐ Regional☐ National☐ Active Duty ☐

3. Who funded this study? (CHECK ALL THAT APPLY)

   VA .... ☐

   DOD .... ☐

   Non-VA/Non-DOD .... ☐

   Not Reported .... ☐

4. Period of service: (CHECK ALL THAT APPLY)

   OEF/OIF ☐   Vietnam ☐   Korea ☐   WW2 ☐
   Persian Gulf/Gulf War ☐   Not Spec. ☐
   Other, specify:_____

5. Topic(s): (CHECK ALL THAT APPLY)

   Clinical research ☐

   Environmental and occupational exposures, post deployment health (military).. ☐

   Non-military exposures.. ☐

   Health behaviors, promotion, prevention, and epidemio-
   logy.. ☐

   Health Services Research

   Education/ training (providers)................................... ☐

   Health status & Health rel. qual. of life .... ☐

   Organizational research .... ☐

   Provider behavior .... ☐

   Quality of care + Patient Satisfaction .... ☐

   Utilization and access .... ☐

   Other .... ☐

   Mortality .... ☐

   Tools (research or clinical) .... ☐

   Vulnerable populations (e.g. homelessness) .... ☐

   Other .... ☐

6. Type of condition(s): (CHECK ALL THAT APPLY)

   Not applicable .... ☐

   Chronic Conditions:

   Bone, join, rheumatic.. ☐

   All vascular disease .... ☐

   Endocrinologic... ☐

   Gastrointestinal .... ☐

   Neurological (includes stroke) .... ☐

   Obesity... ☐

   Thyroid... ☐

   Urologic.. ☐

   Multiple medical conditions...................................... ☐

   Other, specify: .... ☐

   Environmental Exposures .... ☐ ☐

Gender Specific and Reproductive Care:

Benign disease of the female reproductive tract...... ☐

Breast... ☐

Cancers of the reproductive tract .... ☐

Contraception .... ☐

Disease and conditions of pregnancy......................... ☐

Estrogen and Fertility drugs....................................... ☐

STD/STI .... ☐

General gynecological .... ☐

Other, specify: .... ☐

Psychiatric:

Mood Disorders .... ☐

PTSD .... ☐

General psychiatric .... ☐

Other, specify: .... ☐

Substance Abuse:

Alcohol Studies... ☐

Drugs... ☐

Prescription Drugs.. ☐

Smoking.. ☐

General substance abuse .... ☐

Other, specify: .... ☐

Trauma:

MST .... ☐

Polytrauma/TBI/SCI .... ☐

Sexual Assault .... ☐

General Trauma .... ☐

Other, specify: .... ☐

Notes:

APPENDIX 2. STRUCTURED ABSTRACT FORM

Women's Health Structured Abstract

<<CITATION>>
Article ID:

- **Women's health topic areas:**
- **Study Design Category:**
- **Period of Service:**
- **Female Sample Size:**
- **Total Sample Size:**
- **Non patient sample:**
- **Study setting (from where was study population drawn):**

- **Year(s) of study or sampling timeframe:**
- **Purpose of Study:**
- **Outcomes Reported:**

Study design/methods:
- **Study population (active duty, veterans, VAMCs, era, clinic patients, convenience sample, etc):**
- **Women-focused or women as subset population:**
- **Brief Summary of Methods: (describe what was measured, what intervention was performed, what was analyzed and how they did it):**

Main findings:
- **other important items**

APPENDIX 3. SCREENER APPLICATION GUIDELINES

Screener Application Guidelines

Inclusion/Exclusion Criteria: (A) plus at least one of (B), (C), or (D).
- A: If women veterans are convenience sample and being a women veteran is not a unique characteristic for the study, should be STOP
- B: Needs separate results for women or women greater than 75% of the sample. Sex as a covariate does not count unless statistical beta shown.
- C: Study involves active duty military and involves a health condition or functional status that requires medical intervention FOR WOMEN
- D: "Topic is relevant to VA healthcare" TO WOMEN OR "how VA healthcare is delivered " TO WOMEN
- D: If study is not an organizational study and it's only inclusion is because of 1D, then it should be brought to the group for discussion

Study Type:
- Surveys are to be included as observational studies.
- Review articles must have methods section with sufficient detail to replicate to be classified as a systematic review.
- Clinical practice guidelines included under unclear/other.

Sample size:
- List number of women. Also, include full or total sample size.
- For surveys, use the number completed, not the number sent out.
- Identify whether sample is patients or other (e.g., site of care, etc)
  -Determine sample size from analysis, check the n used

Setting:
- Use multi-site if no other option is feasible, VAMC=Hospital, GLA=Integrated HCS

Period of Service:
- Do not use years of military service of study participants (1999, 2002, etc.) to determine period of service. Only identify period if included by article

Topics:
- Every article must have a topic
- For topics, consider access synonymous with availability
- Do not use predictor variables from the analyses to code the study for the screener
- MST/Sexual Assault and similar descriptions are to be categorized under the exposures categories
- Vulnerable populations include: Homeless, transgender, adults with cognitive impairment and SMI (serious mental illness)
- Cognitive behavioral therapy CBT → define as a clinical research topic
- Medication adherence to be categorized as health behavior

Conditions:
- For conditions: only identify those that are a main focus of the article, not adjusters
- Domestic violence should be categorized under General Trauma
- Diabetes should be categorized under Endocrinologic

General note: "grey literature" (theses and other unpublished/ non-peer reviewed works) can be included if they pass the screener's criteria

APPENDIX 4. SEARCH STRATEGY

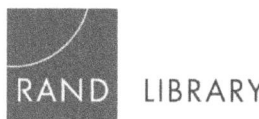

RAND LIBRARY

WOMEN VETERANS HEALTH CARE – SEARCH METHODOLOGY

SEARCH #1

DATABASE SEARCHED & TIME PERIOD COVERED:
PubMed – 2004-8/19/2008

SEARCH STRATEGY:
women* OR gender
AND
veteran*
AND
systematic[sb] OR meta-analysis OR metaanalysis OR women's health services OR quality OR utilization OR patient satisfaction

NUMBER OF RESULTS: 260

SEARCH #2

DATABASE SEARCHED & TIME PERIOD COVERED:
PubMed – 2004-8/19/2008

SEARCH STRATEGY:
"RELATED ARTICLE" SEARCHES ON THE FOLLOWING ARTICLES:
Med Care. 2003 Aug;41(8):950-61.
Gender Differences in service connection for PTSD.
Murdoch M, Hodges J, Hunt C, Cowper D, Kressin N, O'Brien N.

J Gen Intern Med. 2003 Mar;18(3):175-81.
Patient satisfaction in women's clinics versus traditional primary care clinics in the Veterans Administration.
Bean-Mayberry BA, Chang CC, McNeil MA, Whittle J, Hayes PM, Scholle SH.

J Gen Intern Med. 2006 Mar;21 Suppl 3:S11-8.
To use or not to use. What influences why women veterans choose VA health care.
Washington DL, Yano EM, Simon B, Sun S.

J Gen Intern Med. 2006 Mar;21 Suppl 3:S82-92.
The state of women veterans' health research. Results of a systematic literature review.
Goldzweig CL, Balekian TM, Rolón C, Yano EM, Shekelle PG.
AND
systematic[sb] OR meta-analysis OR metaanalysis OR women's health services OR quality OR utilization OR patient satisfaction
AND
women* OR female* OR gender

NUMBER OF RESULTS: 133

SEARCH #3
DATABASE SEARCHED & TIME PERIOD COVERED:
Web of Science SSCI, A&HCI – 2004-9/3/2008

SEARCH STRATEGY:
Topic=(women* OR gender)
AND
Topic=(veteran*)
AND
Topic=(systematic review* OR meta-analysis OR metaanalysis OR health services OR quality OR utilization OR patient satisfaction)

NUMBER OF RESULTS: 140

SEARCH #4

DATABASE SEARCHED & TIME PERIOD COVERED:
Web of Science SSCI, A&HCI – 2004-9/3/2008

SEARCH STRATEGY:
"FORWARD SEARCHES" ON 4 ARTICLES IN SEARCH #2

NUMBER OF RESULTS: 48
NUMBER OF RESULTS BY ARTICLE:
 Med Care. 2003 Aug;41(8):950-61.
Gender Differences in service connection for PTSD.
Murdoch M, Hodges J, Hunt C, Cowper D, Kressin N, O'Brien N.
12

J Gen Intern Med. 2003 Mar;18(3):175-81.
Patient satisfaction in women's clinics versus traditional primary care clinics in the Veterans Administration.
Bean-Mayberry BA, Chang CC, McNeil MA, Whittle J, Hayes PM, Scholle SH.
13

J Gen Intern Med. 2006 Mar;21 Suppl 3:S11-8.
To use or not to use. What influences why women veterans choose VA health care.
Washington DL, Yano EM, Simon B, Sun S.
12

J Gen Intern Med. 2006 Mar;21 Suppl 3:S82-92.
The state of women veterans' health research. Results of a systematic literature review.
Goldzweig CL, Balekian TM, Rolón C, Yano EM, Shekelle PG.
11

SEARCH #5

DATABASE SEARCHED & TIME PERIOD COVERED:
Social Sci Abs, PsycINFO, WorldCat – 2004-9/4/2008

SEARCH STRATEGY:
kw: women* OR kw: gender
AND
kw: veteran*
AND
(kw: systematic and kw: review*) OR kw: meta-analysis OR kw: metaanalysis OR (kw: health and kw: services) OR kw: quality OR kw: utilization OR (kw: patient and kw: satisfaction))

NUMBER OF RESULTS: 176
NUMBER OF RESULTS BY DATABASE: Social Sci Abs (4), PsycINFO (134) WorldCat (42)

APPENDIX 5. DEPLOYMENT AND POST-DEPLOYMENT HEALTH EVIDENCE TABLE

Author	Sample Characteristics	Sample Size	Design/Objective	Main Measures	Main Findings
2007[28]	Female and male service members who deployed to OIF and completed post deployment health assessments (PDHA) and possibly post deployment health reassessments (PDHRA)	Females 23,194 Males 198,989	Observational; To document the frequencies of self-reported symptoms of and provider referrals during PDHAs among service members who subsequently showed evidence of PTSD	Responses to PTSD-related questions of PDHA's and medical referral experiences of Operation Iraqi Freedom (OIF) deployers who were diagnosed with PTSD within six months after return from deployment; and/or screened positive for PTSD on Post Deployment Health Reassessment (PDHRA) questionnaires.	-Among PDHA respondents, 24.9% were referred for health concerns of any type, 10.5% screened positive for PTSD, and 4.1% were referred for mental health concerns. Among PDHA respondents who were clinically diagnosed with PTSD within six months after deployment (n=2676), 54.7% had been referred for a health concern, 48.1% had screened positive for PTSD, and 27.0% had been referred for a mental health concern during their PDHAs. -Females were more likely than males to receive referrals for health concerns in general and for mental health concerns specifically. -However, females were not more likely to screen positive for PTSD during PDHAs. Female and male clinically diagnosed cases and possible cases (per PDHRA responses) of PTSD had a similar prevalence of screening positive for PTSD on their PDHA questionnaire.
2007[21]	Female and male military members who completed deployments for OEF/OIF (n=865674) in 2001-2006	Females 91,424 Males 774,240	Observational; To estimate the natures and incidence of mental disorder-specific diagnoses during medical encounters in the US Military Health System among all recent redeployers from Afghanistan and Iraq.	Natures and incidence of mental disorder-specific diagnoses	1) About 12% of deployers received at least one, and about 5% of deployers received more than one, mental disorder-specific diagnoses after deploying. 2) The demographic subgroups with the highest rates of any mental disorder diagnosis after deploying were females (cumulative incidence: 17.4%), separated/divorced individuals (cumulative incidence: 16.2%), and those of "other" race/ethnicities (cumulative incidence: 15.0%). Deployers who were in the active component, in the Army, younger than 20 years old, and currently or previously married were also significantly more likely than their respective counterparts to receive a mental disorder diagnosis after deployment.

Author	Sample Characteristics	Sample Size	Design/Objective	Main Measures	Main Findings
Adler 2005[33]	U.S. female and male soldiers in non-combat arms units deployed on a NATO peacekeeping mission to the Bosnia area of operations that included Hungary, Bosnia-Herzegovina, and Croatia	Females 1225 Males 2114	Observational; To examine the effects of stressor duration (deployment length) and stressor novelty (no prior deployment experience) on the psychological health of male and female military personnel returning from a peacekeeping deployment	Correlations between demographics, deployment experience, and dependent variables by gender; length of deployment and mean scale score of depressive and posttraumatic stress symptoms by gender; deployment experience and mean scale score of depressive and posttraumatic stress symptoms by gender	Longer deployments and 1st-time deployments were associated with an increase in distress scores. However, the relationship between deployment length and increased distress was found only for male soldiers.
Araneta 2004[41]	Military women who were admitted to military hospitals for pregnancy-related diagnoses between August 2, 1990 and May 31, 1992	Females 1110	Observational; (1) To enumerate Gulf-War (GW) exposed conceptions (2) characterize reproductive outcomes among GW-exposed conceptions and (3) to compare reproductive outcomes of GW-exposed pregnancies with postwar conceptions of women GW veterans and women nondeployed veterans who belonged to deployed units.	The number of pregnancies, number of postwar conceptions (both deployed and nondeployed), similarity of adverse reproductive outcomes, number of spontaneous abortions and ectopic pregnancies	Gulf War-exposed conceptions and nondeployed conceptions had similar outcomes. However, GW veteran postwar conceptions were at increased risk for ectopic pregnancies and spontaneous abortions.

Author	Sample Characteristics	Sample Size	Design/Objective	Main Measures	Main Findings
Cavin 2005[36]	Case series of 12 World War II spies	Females 5 Males 7	Observational; To discover if there were two types of soldiers: those who never talked about the war and those who could not stop talking about it.	Discussion of PTSD symptoms and wartime excitement	1) Three of 12 still had PTSD symptoms nearly 50 years later. Many of these veterans constantly talked about their war-time experience throughout adult life. 2) The majority of the 12, regardless of gender, still exhibited war excitement when discussing their roles in the war. For 11 of 12, they were still visibly excited by war talk. For 10 of 12, war bonding evoked more powerful feelings than subsequent social relationships. 3) This case series of interviews related to PTSD was unique because it was a mixed gender cohort; it includes men and women with the same stressors; the women in the OSS study are not sexual victims; the research focuses on high functioning vets; it differs from a focus on combat soldiers; and it is derived from sociological interviews, not medical studies.
Erbes 2007[15]	Female and male OEF/OIF veteran enrollees (n=120) at one Midwestern VAMC who had returned within a six-month time frame, agreed to participate and completed a questionnaire	Females 17 Males 103	Observational; To evaluate levels of PTSD, depression, alcohol abuse, and the associations with quality of life, and mental health service utilization among returnees from OEF/OIF.	Psychiatric distress levels (measured by PTSD symptoms, depression symptoms, and hazardous alcohol use), functional impairment, and service utilization	1) PTSD levels (12%) were consistent with previous research while problematic drinking levels were also elevated (33%). 2) PTSD and alcohol abuse were associated with lower quality of life in multiple domains, even when controlling for depression. 3) Of those screening positive for PTSD, 56% reported using mental health services. Only 18% of those screening positive for alcohol abuse reported using such services. 4) No reported findings were identified as related to gender.

Author	Sample Characteristics	Sample Size	Design/Objective	Main Measures	Main Findings
Farley 2006[29]	Female soldiers seen at the 325th Combat Support Hospital (CSH; Bagram Air force Base, Afghanistan)	Females 62	Observational; To evaluate the value, unit cost, and medical effectiveness of providing specialized obstetric and gynecological care "far forward", at echelon III [the combat support hospital (CSH)] in the operating theatre of Afghanistan during OEF, rotation 5.	Total # of female patient seen at the CSH, average distance traveled for treatment, mean travel times, time to appointment, and woman-hours lost from each unit	A total of 62 cases were seen at the CSH, where 57 total patients were seen at the CSH (echelon III) and 5 were sent to Germany for care (echelon IV or V). 88% of the soldiers seen were of enlisted rank, 9% were officers, and 3% were civilians. Three (60%) of the patients sent to Germany were of enlisted rank, 1 (20%) was of officer rank, and 1 (20%) was a civilian employee. The military unit branch of origin varied greatly. 7% of the patients seen at the CSH were seen for their annual well-woman examination, 68% for abnormal cervical cytology and colposcopies, and 25% for other conditions (including pregnancy, dysfunctional uterine bleeding, and pelvic pain). The majority of the patients seen at the CSH were from BAF. The average distance traveled ($p<0.0001$), mean travel time ($p<0.0035$), time to appointment ($p<0.035$), and total time lost from each unit was significantly different for those traveling to Germany versus the CSH.
Felker 2008[11]	Female and male military service members presenting to a mental health clinic in Kuwait	Females 78 Males 214	Observational; To (1) describe the feasibility of using well-validated, screening measures, and (2) describe demographic and clinical characteristics of a sample of OIF military personnel who sought mental health care while deployed.	PTSD assessment; depression, alcohol use disorders and life stressors	-A total of 19% of the sample subjects screened positive for post-traumatic stress disorder-related symptoms, 35% for a major depressive disorder, and 11% for severe misuse of alcohol. Significant levels of distress and functional impairment were reported by 58% of the sample. -Women represented a disproportionately high percentage of those presenting for care (27%). Female service members might represent a high-risk group.

Systematic Review of Women Veterans Health Research 2004-2008

Author	Sample Characteristics	Sample Size	Design/Objective	Main Measures	Main Findings
Haas 2007[32]	All women presenting to the obstetrics clinic for prenatal care appointments at Naval Hospital Camp Lejeune from Jan to Apr 2005	Females 463	Observational; To determine if having a partner deployed in the military during wartime increased the stress levels in pregnant women and to determine predictors of reporting higher stress	Relationship between having a deployed partner and stress levels in pregnant women	Over 88.2% of patients responded to the survey. Women with deployed partners more often reported higher stress levels than those with homeland partners (39.6% and 24.2%, respectively; p<0.01). Logistic regression revealed that having a partner deployed (OR 1.89, 95% CI 1.00-3.57, p=0.04), being active duty (OR 2.64, 95% CI 1.43-4.87, p=<0.01), advanced gestational age (OR 1.04, 95% CI 1.00-1.07, p=0.03) and having >1child at home (OR 2.30, 95% CI 1.12-4.73, p=0.02) all predicted higher stress reporting. Having a support person present was protective against stress (OR 0.40, 95% CI 0.20-0.78, p=<0.01).
Helmer 2007[14]	Female and male veteran convenience sample from OEF/OIF active duty and reserve components (n=56) who were clinic patients at one War Related Illness and Injury Center (WRIISC)	Females 11 Males 45	Observational (retrospective chart review); To describe the health and exposure concerns of a clinical case series of OEF/OIF veterans and compare findings between active duty and reserve components.	Physical health concerns (e.g., genito-urinary concerns), exposure concerns (e.g., depleted uranium, multiple vaccinations, and poor air quality from burning trash), mental health concerns (e.g., PTSD)	1) Compared to reserve veterans, most active duty veterans were male, single, and young. 2) Environmental exposure concern specific to the burning of trash and feces was higher among reserve veterans (43.6% vs. 11.8%; p=.02). 3) Physical and mental health concerns were similar between the two groups. 4) A comparison of genitourinary concerns between men (80% of our case series) and women (20% of our case series) did not demonstrate a significant difference by gender.
Hoge 2007[13]	Female and male Iraq veterans, from four Army combat infantry brigades, surveyed 1 year after their return from deployment	Females 80 Males 2783	Observational; This study evaluated the association of PTSD with physical health measures among Iraq war veterans 1 year after their return from deployment with control for combat injury.	Past month symptoms of PTSD, depression, alcohol misuse, self-rated health status, sick call visits, missed work days, and somatic symptoms.	-Among all participants, 16.6% met screening criteria for PTSD. PTSD was significantly associated with lower ratings of general health, more sick call visits, more missed workdays, more physical symptoms, and high somatic symptom severity. These results remained significant after controlling for being wounded or injured. -The high prevalence of PTSD and its strong association with physical health problems among Iraq war veterans have important implications for delivery of medical services. The medical burden of PTSD includes physical health problems; combat veterans with serious somatic concerns should be evaluated for PTSD.

Author	Sample Characteristics	Sample Size	Design/Objective	Main Measures	Main Findings
Hoge 2006[20]	Female and male Army soldiers and marines who completed a Post-Deployment Health Assessment (PDHA) on return from deployments to OEF/OIF) and other locations (eg., Bosnia, Kosovo)	Females 32,500 Males 271404	Observational; To determine the relationship between deployment to Iraq and Afghanistan and mental health care utilization during the first year after return and to evaluate lessons learned from the postemployment mental health screening effort, particularly the correlation between screening results and actual use of mental health services.	Screening positive for PTSD, major depression, or other mental health problems; referral for a mental health reason; use of mental health care services after returning from deployment; attrition from military services	1) The prevalence rates of mental health problems and combat experiences were consistently higher following deployment to OIF than to OEF or other locations. Among OIF veterans, 23.6% of women reported a mental health concern compared with 18.6% of men. 2) Referral to mental health was strongly correlated with screening positive for a mental health problem on the PDHA. Hospitalization was significantly associated with deployment location and reporting a mental health concern on the PDHA. (3) OIF veterans used impatient and outpatient mental health services at higher rates after deployment than OEF veterans and service members who deployed to other locations.
Hoge 2004[17]	Female and male OEF/OIF active duty military from 4 combat units (Army or Marine)	Females 63 Males 6117	Observational; To (1) study the prevalence of mental health problems among members of the military personnel recruited from combat units before or after their deployment to Iraq or Afghanistan, and (2) identify the proportion of service members with mental health concerns who were not receiving care and the barriers perceived to accessing and receiving care.	Symptoms in the past month of major depressive disorder, generalized anxiety disorder, and PTSD; current stress, emotional problems, alcohol problems, or family problems; use of mental health services in past month or year; perceived barriers to use	-Military personnel returning from Iraq were more likely to report a mental health problem, interest in receiving help, and use of mental health services. -Rates of PTSD were significantly higher after combat duty in Iraq than before deployment. Significant associations were reported for major depression the misuse of alcohol.

Author	Sample Characteristics	Sample Size	Design/Objective	Main Measures	Main Findings
Katz 2007[16]	Female OEF/OIF veterans who were referred to a single Women's Mental Health Center for individual psychotherapy	Females 18	Observational; To determine whether: (1) women have increased emotional symptoms because of difficulties readjusting to civilian life and (2) women have a unique experience in war compared with their male counterparts.	clinician symptom rating; Military Sexual Trauma (MST); being injured in Iraq; witnessing others injured or killed; and relationships between readjustment, symptoms, and events	-Women who had MST had more symptoms and more difficulties with readjustment to civilian life than those without MST.
Lambert 2006[26]	Female and males forming a case series	Females 1 Males 4	Observational; To report a series of consecutive cases of PTSD affected combat veterans who were treated with the atypical antipsychotic agent aripiprazole (i.e., Abilify)	Sleep disturbances, nightmares, anxiety in crowds	The five cases combat-related PTSD treated with aripiprazole and either sertraline or cognitive-behavioral psychotherapy illustrate a significant improvement, but not total resolution of symptoms in most cases.
Lapierre 2007[22]	Female and male active duty soldiers, who participated in a reintegration training program after returning from Iraq or Afghanistan	Females 263 Males 3826	Observational; To identify rates of posttraumatic stress and depressive symptoms in soldiers returning from war	Self-reported levels of depressions, posttraumatic stress, and life satisfaction	1) Women comprised only a small sample (6%). 2) After deployment, about 44% of study participants reported clinically significant depressive and/or posttraumatic stress symptoms. Soldiers returning from Iraq reported somewhat more mental health problems and treatment seeking than soldiers returning from Afghanistan. 3) Being separated or divorced (vs. married) was associated with increased reports of posttraumatic stress and depressive symptoms. Compared to NCOs and officers, junior enlisted soldiers reported more posttraumatic and depressive symptoms. 4) Female participants were more likely to report depressive symptoms; however, gender was not a predictor for posttraumatic stress symptoms for either sample (OIF and OEF). 5) Soldiers seek help for the symptoms; however, only 16% of OIF participants and 13% of OEF participants with symptoms did so.

60

Author	Sample Characteristics	Sample Size	Design/Objective	Main Measures	Main Findings
Lindstrom 2006[35]	Active-duty enlisted Navy and Marine Corps females in combat support and noncombat support occupations	Females 73,777	Observational; To conduct an exploratory study to develop a baseline assessment of the mental health hospitalization rates of military women working in newly gender-integrated combat support occupations prior to the onset of the wars in Iraq and Afghanistan	Relationship between number of hospitalizations in combat and noncombat support and mental disorders (e.g, substance abuse disorders, adjustment disorders, mood disorders, etc).	Using Cox regression to adjust for all variables in the model, results indicated that women working in combat support occupations were less likely (HR 0.64, 95% CI 0.53–0.77) to be hospitalized for a mental illness compared with women working in noncombat support occupations. The study also reported that older women were slightly more likely to have a mental health hospitalization (HR 1.21, 95% CI 1.04–1.41) compared with women in the youngest age category, ≤19 years. Additionally, white women were significantly more likely to have a mental health hospitalization when compared with black women (HR 1.41, 95% CI 1.24–1.60).
McNulty 2005[25]	Female and male active duty Navy service members deployed on aircraft carriers during OEF/OIF in 2002-2003	Females 259 Males 1182	Observational; To describe the healthcare needs and perceived stressors of active duty members deployed to Iraq during the predeployment, middeployment, and postdeployment phases. Stress & HC needs during Navy deploy	Member well-being, adaptation, coping, anxiety, stress, and health care needs	Many variables predicted extreme anxiety during deployment, including middeployment phase, age under 25 years, being childless, nonattendance at church, being enlisted, zero- or one-deployment history; no high school education, and being currently in counseling. Active duty members in all phases of deployment had equally disturbing levels of anxiety. All phases reported suicidal ideation at alarming rates (2.4% in predeployment, 4.9% in mid-deployment, and 3% in postdeployment).
Pierce 1999[42]	Stratified, random sample of US Air Force military women selected from a Department of Defense database who served in Operation Desert Shield or Desert Storm	Females 525	Observational; To provide baseline health information on a randomized sample of military women serving during the Persian Gulf War.	Prevalence of gender specific health problems, rate of health care utilization, satisfaction with military and civilian care during respondents' military careers	-The most prevalent gender-specific problems were problems during pregnancy (41%), urinary tract infection (34%), headache (33%), and menstrual irregularities (32%) and abnormal Pap smear (27%). - Of note, many women did not seek health care for their problems. -In this overall group, 76% reported using military health care, 41% used civilian health care, and only 3% reported using the VA for care. -Overall, for 15 of 18 conditions, satisfaction ratings were higher for civilian care.

61

Author	Sample Characteristics	Sample Size	Design/Objective	Main Measures	Main Findings
Pierce 1997[39]	Stratified, random sample of US Air Force military women selected from a Department of Defense database who served in Operation Desert Shield or Desert Storm	Females 525	Observational; To describe the effects of deployment and military service during the Persian Gulf war on women's physical and emotional health	General physical health, gender specific and reproductive health, 18 symptoms of gender-specific health problems, subscales for anxiety, depression, somatization, and PTSD	Women deployed to theatre reported significantly more general as well as gender-specific health problems than did women deployed elsewhere. A cluster of common health problems included: skin rash; cough; depression; unintentional weight loss; insomnia; and memory problems. Women serving in theatre also reported a significant increase in several gender-specific problems compared to women deployed elsewhere.
Rundell 2006[19]	Female and male OEF/OIF active duty military evacuated from theatre due to psychiatric conditions (n=1264)	Females 237 Males 1027	Observational; To characterize the demographic composition, clinical diagnoses and clinical dispositions given to OEF/OIF psychiatric patients seen at the Landstuhl Regional Medical Center (LRMC).	Demographic information, clinical diagnosis, and clinical dispositions for the LRMC OEF/OIF psychiatric patients	1) Psychiatric evacuees were more likely to be female, African-American of Hispanic, under the age of 31 years, enlisted and National Guard Reserve, as opposed to active-duty military. 2) More than 80% of patients were evacuated during the first 6 months, compared with only 17% during the second 6 months of deployment; less than 5% of the LRMC psychiatric evacuees were returned to OEF/OIF duty. 3) Women were overrepresented as psychiatric evacuees almost by a factor 2, which suggests the possibility that there are gender-specific risks that increase the possibility of becoming a psychiatric evacuee.

Author	Sample Characteristics	Sample Size	Design/Objective	Main Measures	Main Findings
Seal 2008[24]	Female and male veterans with military separation dates after September 11, 2001 presenting for care at one VA medical center or its community based clinics	Females 83 Males 750	Observational; To determine the frequency and predictors of implementation of the VA postdeployment screen; the proportion of veterans with positive screens for PTSD, depression or high risk alcohol use; the proportion of veterans seen in a VA mental health clinic within 90 days and beyond	PTSD screen, depression, alcohol use, and completion of a mental health appointment for those screening positive	Postdeployment screening was more likely in veterans who had a primary care visit versus other settings (72% vs 12%; adjusted odds ratio [AOR]=13.3; 95% confidence interval [CI]=8.31, 21.3) and for those seen at a VA community clinic rather than at the medical center (87% vs 37%; AOR=3.56; 95% CI=1.78, 7.11). African American veterans of OIF or OEF were less likely to be screened than were White veterans (29% vs 49%; AOR=0.45; 95% CI=0.22, 0.91). The likelihood of a follow-up mental health visit within 90 days of screening was increased for veterans who were seen in a VA community clinic versus the medical center (AOR=6.08; 95% CI=1.56, 23.6) and for those seen in primary care versus another outpatient setting (AOR=19.4; 95% CI=1.30, 290).
Seal 2007[12]	Female and male veterans, serving in OEF/OIF, and new users of VA health care system	Females 13,652 Males 90,117	Observational; To (1) describe the proportion of OEF/OIF veterans seen in VA facilities who received one or more mental health and/or psychosocial diagnoses and the timing and clinical setting of first mental health diagnoses, and (2) identify subgroups of OEF/OIF veteransat high risk for receiving mental health diagnoses after returning from military service.	Mental health diagnoses and psychosocial problems	Of 103,788 OEF/OIF/OIF veterans first seen at VA health care facilities following OEF/OIF service, a quarter received mental health diagnoses, and more than half of these veterans were dually or multiply diagnosed. The most common military service–related mental health diagnosis was PTSD. When psychosocial problems were considered, overall, nearly a third of OEF/OIF veterans were classified as having either mental health diagnoses and/or psychosocial problems. Of veterans receiving mental health diagnoses, the majority were diagnosed on or within days of their first VA clinic visit. Most initial mental health diagnoses occurred in non-mental health settings, particularly in primary care settings. Minimal absolute differences were found between

Author	Sample Characteristics	Sample Size	Design/Objective	Main Measures	Main Findings
Smith 2008[10]	Female and male military service members previously deployed to Iraq and Afghanistan, exposed to combat, who had no PTSD at baseline assessment	Females 890 Males 4469	Observational; To conduct a prospective investigation of the relationship between prior assault and PTSD in a military cohort deployed to combat in Iraq and Afghanistan.	PTSD assessment, assault history, assault history, behavioral risk factors, and combat exposure.	-New-onset PTSD symptoms or diagnosis among deployed military reporting combat exposures occurred in 22% of women who reported prior assault and 10% not reporting prior assault. -Among men reporting prior assault, rates were 12% and 6%, respectively. -Adjusting for baseline factors, the odds of new-onset PTSD symptoms was more than 2-fold higher in both women and men who reported assault prior to deployment.
Smith 2008[23]	Female and male active duty military enrolled in the Millenium Cohort Study surveyed before and after the wars in Iraq and Afghanistan	Females 13849 Males 36279	Observational; To investigate prospectively the effect of military deployment and self reported exposure to combat on new onset and persistent symptoms of PTSD in a large population based military cohort	Self-reported PTSD symptoms (PCL-C);	Over 40% of the cohort was deployed between 2001 and 2006; 24% deployed for the first time in support of the wars in Iraq and Afghanistan. Incidence rates of 10-13 cases of PTSD per 1000 person years occurred in the millennium cohort. New onset self reported PTSD symptoms or diagnosis were identified in 7.6-8.7% of deployers who reported combat exposures, 1.4-2.1% of deployers who did not report combat exposures, and 2.3-3.0% of nondeployers.
Smith 2007[38]	Large, longitudinal, population-based cohort of active duty military servicemen and women with oversample of those recently deployed, female or reserve/guard members.	Females 20106 Males 75413	Observational; To evaluate the baseline functional health status of a large population-based military cohort	Physical and mental health component scores (PCS and MCS) of the SF36-V	-The baseline physical and mental health component scores of a military cohort is slightly more favorable than that of the same-age, same-sex U.S. general population. -Factors associated with more favorable health status were male gender, marriage, higher education, higher military rank, and Air Force service. Combat specialists had similar health status compared to other military occupations. -Gender-specific results showed increasing age was associated with more favorable MCS scores and less favorable PCS scores among active duty and reserve/guard women. Similar results were found among men.

Author	Sample Characteristics	Sample Size	Design/Objective	Main Measures	Main Findings
Smith 2007[40]	Subset of female responders to the Millennium Cohort questionnaire (derived from all US Military personnel serving in October 2000)	Females 20139	Observational; (1) To establish the degree of concordance between self-reported occupation and the electronically maintained personnel occupation data. (2) To describe occupational exposures among a current cohort of US military women.	(1) The reliability of self-reported occupation when compared with electronically maintained data; (2) odds of women in certain occupations (adjusting for demographic and military characteristics) to report particular exposures of concern (potentially toxic environmental exposures or disturbing experiences)	-Self-reported occupations were moderate to highly reliable when compared to electronic data. Health care specialists demonstrated almost perfect agreement, and trainees demonstrated poor agreement. -Occupation, age, education, pay grade, and service branch were significantly associated with reporting witnessing death, witnessing trauma, exposure to chemical or biological warfare, exposure to depleted uranium, and exposure to pesticides. (p<0.05) -After adjustment for demographic and military factors, deployment to SW Asia, Bosnia, or Kosovo (from 1998-2000), and deployment to the 1991 Gulf War, active-duty women health care specialists were significantly more likely to report witnessing death or trauma compared to combat specialists. -Active-duty women specialists in the field of electrical/mechanical equipment repair were significantly more likely to report witnessing death, exposure to depleted uranium, and pesticides compared with combat specialists.
Stecker 2007[27]	Female and male National Guard soldiers who had served in OIF and screened positive for 1 or more mental health disorders	Females 2 Males 20	Observational; To assess beliefs about mental health treatment in a group of soldiers newly returning from Iraq.	Seeking mental health treatment after returning from Iraq; normative and control beliefs about mental health treatment	Stigma was portrayed as a major disadvantage to treatment seeking. Yet most participants indicated that people would be supportive of treatment seeking. Reducing symptoms was a major advantage to care. Barriers included pride, not being able to ask for help, and not being able to admit to having a problem.
Stetz 2005[18]	Female and male soldiers medically evacuated from theatre due to psychiatric conditions (n=5671; with 9% missing gender)	Females 912 Males 4264	Observational; To present a snapshot of the main psychiatric reasons reported for medevacs during OEF/OIF.	Medevac cases from OEF and OIF; psychiatric diagnoses with ICD-9 codes; gender; military rank	Psychiatric diagnoses were the 2nd leading cause of medevacs in OEF and 4th leading cause in OIF. For medevacs from OEF, 18% of the troops were women, while in OIF, 16% of troops were female. The proportion of medevacs with psychiatric diagnoses by gender was 33% women for OEF and 17% women for OIF.

Author	Sample Characteristics	Sample Size	Design/Objective	Main Measures	Main Findings
Thomson 2006[30]	Female active, reserve and National Guard units deployed in Iraq or Kuwait for at least 3 months, but no more than 8 months	Females 251	Observational; To assess women's perceptions of health care delivery in OIF, specifically those receiving care at the echelon I and II level (front line and aid station).	predeployment screening, contraceptive method availability and side effects, accessibility of gynecological care, field hygiene counseling, and smoking status	All respondents were of reproductive age, except two. Irregular bleeding was the most common side effect among soldiers using hormonal contraception. Ortho Evra patches fell off in 58% of cases, 23% of soldiers changed contraceptive methods once they were in the field because of unavailability of their previous method, 21% of soldiers experienced some type of gynecological problems, and 44% could not access gynecological care. 26% of soldiers received predeployment menstrual hygiene counseling, and of those, 77% attempting cycle control succeeded. Almost one half of the respondents did not meet the cervical cytological screening practice guidelines supported by the American College of Obstetricians and Gynecologists.
Vogt 2008[31]	Female and male active duty service members deployed to Iraq	Females 49 Males 640	Observational; validation study; To validate 9 scales from the Deployment Risk and Resilience Inventory (DRRI) in a large sample of Operation Iraqi Freedom (OIF) army personnel diversified in occupational and demographic characteristics.	Reliability and validity of DRRI scales	Evidence for internal consistency reliability was quite strong and similar to that demonstrated in a sample of Gulf War I veterans on which these scales were originally developed and validated. In general, DRRI scales demonstrated reasonable to excellent values for coefficient alpha, suggesting that the item sets converged on a common construct. Significant gender differences emerged for 5 of the variables. Men reported greater exposure to combat and aftermath of battle and more often reported being well prepared for deployment. Women reported greater perceived threat compared to men.

Author	Sample Characteristics	Sample Size	Design/Objective	Main Measures	Main Findings
Vogt 2005[34]	National sample of Gulf War I female and male veterans identified through the Manpower Data Center and VA Gulf War Health Registry, with an overrepresentation of women (25% women, 75% men) and representations from all branches of the military	Females 83 Males 233	Observational; To examine deployment stressors to elucidate gender differences in war-zone exposure and identify gender-based differential associations between stressors and mental health outcomes.	Mission related stressors, interpersonal stressors, mental health outcomes (depression, anxiety, posttraumatic stress (PTSD) symptomatology)	The response rate was 66%, and women were slightly less likely to participate than men (56% vs. 67%). As deployment social support decreased, levels of depression increased for both women and men. However, the depression slope was much steeper for women. As levels of sexual harassment increased, levels of depression or anxiety increased sharply for men, and changed very little for women, possibly representing a stronger risk factor for men. For anxiety levels, both concerns about family disruptions and lack of deployment social support resulted in higher anxiety, especially for women.
Wolfe 1992[37]	National sample of Vietnam veteran females who had participated in research conducted at the National Center for Post-Traumatic Stress Disorder.	Females 76	Observational; To examine the status of PTSD in a cohort of women after the onset of Operation Desert Storm.	Changes in PTSD symptoms (in particular; re-experiencing, avoidance/ numbing, and hyperarousal), and ratings on a series of broad-based psychological symptoms (SCL-90-R).	One-way ANOVAs indicated that the group of female veterans who had previously reported high levels of PTSD were significantly more susceptible to greater distress across all three PTSD ratings (p<0.001). Univariate tests showed significant differences between the two groups on all nine dimensions of the SCL-90-R, (p<0.005).

APPENDIX 6. ORGANIZATIONAL RESEARCH EVIDENCE TABLE

Author	Sample Characteristics	Sample Size	Design/Objective	Main Measures	Main Findings
Bean-Mayberry 2007[43]	National sample of VA sites serving 4,000 or more unique patients and delivering 20,000 or more outpatient visits in fiscal year 1998	VA sites 155	Observational; To understand organizational influences on the development of women's health clinics for primary care delivery in VA facilities.	Proportion of VA Medical Centers with established women's health clinics (WHC) for primary care (PC); organizational factors associated with presence of WHCs for primary care	-133 VA Medical centers (61%) have established WHCs for Primary Care. -The majority of WHCs providing PC services were at VAMCs (103 of 160; 64%) compared to CBOCs (30 of 59; 51%). -The only factor significantly associated with established WHCs for PC was separate primary care leadership (OR 3.62, 95%CI 1.45- 9.05).
Bean-Mayberry 2007[45]	Original Comprehensive VA Women's Health Centers and Department of Health and Human Services (DHHS) National Centers of Excellence in Women's Health	VA sites 8 DHHS sites 13	Observational; To assess and contrast the features of prototypical women's centers in VA and DHHS	Comparison of organizational structure of comprehensive women's health centers categorized by diffusion theory – system openness, centralization, complexity, formalization, interconnectedness and organizational slack	-All DHHS and VA centers served urban areas, and nearly all had academic partnerships. DHHS centers had three times the average caseload as VA centers. -Preventive cancer screening and general reproductive services were uniformly available at all centers, although DHHS centers offered more extensive reproductive services on-site more frequently, and VA centers more often had on-site mental health care. -The DHHS and VA sites were similar in complexity (training or fellowship programs), formalization (quality monitoring activities), interconnectedness (programs for training other providers in women's health), and organizational slack (extended/weekend hours or same gender providers).
Cope 2006[47]	National sample of VA sites serving at least 400 or more women veterans in fiscal year 2000	VA sites 126	Observational; To describe the variation in provision of hormonal and intrauterine contraception among Veterans Affairs (VA) facilities.	Provision of 2 contraceptive services: 1) prescription and management of hormonal contraception; and 2) IUD placement	-97 percent of facilities offered onsite prescription and management of hormonal contraception and 60% offered IUD placement. -Three organizational factors were independently associated with onsite IUD placements: onsite gynecologist (OR 20.35, 95% CI 7.02-58.74); hospital-based in contrast to community-based practice (OR 5.49, 95% CI 1.16-26.10); and availability of a clinician providing women's health training to other clinicians (OR 3.40 95% CI 1.19-9.76).

Author	Sample Characteristics	Sample Size	Design/Objective	Main Measures	Main Findings
Hall 2007[48]	Sample of military sexual trauma (MST) health providers at sites in one VA regional network	VA MST Providers 34	Observational; To measure identified factors in the MST practice environment that influence delivery of care and measure levels of perceived organizational support among MST providers	Individual, facility and regional military sexual trauma practice environment (MST-PE) variable scores and levels of perceived organizational support (POS) were calculated	-All four independent variables and four of five descriptive variables were significantly correlated with POS (p<.01 for each comparison). Scheduling was significant at p<.05. -Ethical conflicts, burnout, vicarious trauma, and isolation had negative correlations with the POS while workload, organizational culture, leadership, and MST resources were positively correlated with POS. -Wide variability existed between facilities on the POS instrument, even with the small sample size.
Seelig 2008[44]	National sample of VA sites serving 400 or more women veterans in fiscal year 2000	VA Sites 136	Observational; To assess the availability of basic and advanced GYN services by clinic type and staffing arrangements	Availability of GYN services by clinic type; availability of advanced GYN services by presence of OB-GYN physician or GYN clinic	-Basic gynecologic services had widespread availability across nearly all sites. -Sites were more likely to have all five advanced gynecologic services when an OBGYN physician was routinely available (p<.01 for each service) and were more likely to have endometrial biopsy and IUD insertion when a GYN clinic was available (p<.01 for each service).
Washington 2006[46]	National sample of VA sites serving 400 or more women veterans in fiscal year 2000	VA Sites 118	Observational; To assess the availability of women's health care specialists for emergency gynecological problems (GYN) and for emergency mental health conditions specific to women (WMH).	Availability of women's health care specialists for emergency gynecologic problems (GYN) and emergency mental health (MH) conditions specific to women during clinic hours and after hours.	-The majority of sites had GYN and MH specialists available for emergencies during clinic hours (64.4% and 82.7% of sites, respectively). -Availability of specialists after hours for GYN emergencies was 39.8%, for MH emergencies was 51.7%. -Two significant predictors: separate women's health clinic was associated with availability of emergency GYN services (beta: 0.279, p=0.023), and lower local managed care penetration was associated with availability of emergency MH conditions specific to women (beta: -0.282, p=0.024).

Author	Sample Characteristics	Sample Size	Design/Objective	Main Measures	Main Findings
Yano 2006[49]	National sample of VA sites serving 400 or more women veterans with a women's health clinic (WHCs; n=66) compared to the original 8 VA Comprehensive Women's Health Centers (CWHCs)	VA Sites 74	Observational; To assess the degree to which VA medical centers WHCs compare to the original CWHC model programs.	Organizational features categorized by innovative organizational domains such as centralization (budget control), complexity (scope of services), formalization (procedures), interconnectedness (WH leadership on committees), organizational slack (budget changes, staffing), size, and system openness (academic affiliation).	- Gender-specific service availability in WHCs was comparable to that of CWHCs with important exceptions in mental health, mammography and osteoporosis management. -WHCs were less likely to have same-gender providers ($p < .05$), women's health training programs ($p < .01$), separate women's mental health clinics ($p < .001$), separate space ($p < .05$), or adequate privacy ($p < .05$); however, they were less likely to have experienced educational program closures ($p < .001$) and staffing losses ($p < .05$) compared to CWHCs.

APPENDIX 7. QUALITY OF CARE EVIDENCE TABLE

Author	Sample Characteristics	Sample Size	Design/Objective	Main Measures	Main Findings
2007[90]	Females younger than age 50 who served in the active component of the US Armed Forces anytime between Jan 2005 and June 2006	Females 117110	Observational; To document prescriptions for hormonal contraceptives available through military medical facilities	Percentage of the surveillance population younger than age 50 who filled one or more prescriptions for hormonal contraceptives during a 27-month period	Hormonal contraceptive prescriptions were filled for more than half (54.2%) of all females who served in the active US military. The majority of females who were prescribed hormonal contraceptives were <25 years old (51.2%), white (55%), and not married (56.7%). Females in their twenties were more likely than those younger or older to receive prescriptions for hormonal contraceptives – overall and for each type except the IUD with progestin.
Albright 2005[84]	Active duty female soldiers presenting at an Army Medical Center or clinic with dysuria or vaginal symptoms	Females 238	Observational; To identify whether specific behavior patterns (e.g., fluid restriction, use of mechanical devices, and postponement of voiding) were associated with dysuria.	Voiding frequency during day or night and behaviors associated with dysuria	Voiding frequency was lower during day or night in the field for women with dysuria. More women in dysuria group reported fluid restriction; were treated for dysuria in the field or after field duty; and used tampons, pads or devices to control urinary incontinence during field duty. More women with dysuria postponed voiding during field or regular duty.
Araneta 2004[41]	Military women who were admitted to military hospitals for pregnancy-related diagnoses between August 2, 1990 and May 31, 1992	Females 1110	Observational; (1) To enumerate Gulf-War (GW) exposed conceptions and (2) characterize reproductive outcomes among GW-exposed conceptions and (3) to compare reproductive outcomes of GW-exposed pregnancies with postwar conceptions of women GW veterans and women nondeployed veterans who belonged to deployed units.	The number of pregnancies, number of postwar conceptions (both deployed and nondeployed), similarity of adverse reproductive outcomes, number of spontaneous abortions and ectopic pregnancies	Gulf War-exposed conceptions and nondeployed conceptions had similar outcomes. However, GW veteran postwar conceptions were at increased risk for ectopic pregnancies and spontaneous abortions.

Author	Sample Characteristics	Sample Size	Design/Objective	Main Measures	Main Findings
Barnard 2003[82]	National sample of female veterans who had at least 1 visit between July 1, 1994 and June 30, 1995, and were still menstruating	Females 1736	Observational; To assess the prevalence of menstrual symptoms and the degree to which these symptoms affect health status, by comparing women with and without menstrual symptoms.	All eight domains of short form (SF-36) health status survey	Of the 1744 menstruating women, 67% answered yes to at least one of the 3 items relating to menstrual symptoms. Women with menstrual symptoms had significantly lower scores for all domains of the SF-36 (p<.01), except energy and vitality (p<.05), both before and after adjustment for sociodemographic, psychosocial, and comorbidity variables. Results remained unchanged when the analyses were repeated and limited only to women without a depression or a sexual trauma history.
Barnett 2006[75]	Male and female veterans and nonveterans in VA and Medicare HMOs	VA Females 3311 VA Males 120,322 Non-VA Females 88,970 Non-VA Males 68,547	Observational; To determine if rates of inappropriate medication use in the elderly differ between the VA health care system and the private sector Medicare health maintenance organization (HMO) patients.	Rate of inappropriate prescribing in the elderly VA and Medicare patients	1) Compared with private sector patients, VA patients were less likely to receive any inappropriate medication overall (21% vs. 29%, p<0.001), and in each classification: always avoid (2% vs. 5% p<0.001), rarely appropriate (8% vs. 13%, p<0.001), and some indications (15% vs. 17%, p<0.001). 2) The rate of inappropriate drug use was lower in the VA compared with the private sector for males (21% vs. 24% p<0.001) and females (28% vs. 32%, p<0.001).
Bean-Mayberry 2006[50]	Random sample of female veterans using VA primary care or women's clinics across 5 states	Females 1447	Observational; To explore effect of race on primary care quality and satisfaction among women in the VA	4 domains of primary care delivery: patient preference for provider; interpersonal communication; accumulated knowledge; and coordination of care	-Race had no association with any of the 4 primary care domains or overall satisfaction. Gynecological care from VA provider was associated with perfect ratings on patient preference for provider (OR 2.0, 95% CI 1.3, 3.1) and satisfaction (OR 1.6, 95% CI 1.2, 2.3), while female provider was associated with interpersonal communication (OR 1.9, 95% CI 1.4, 2.6).

Author	Sample Characteristics	Sample Size	Design/Objective	Main Measures	Main Findings
Bean-Mayberry 2006[54]	Female veterans in women's clinics or primary care clinics at 10 VA medical centers in one region	Females 1080	Observational; To determine whether separate or combined effects of provider gender, availability of gynecologic services from the provider, and women's clinic setting improve patient ratings of primary care.	Patient perceptions of primary care were measured using the validated 19-item Components of Primary Care Index (CPCI) which consists of 4 multi-item primary care domains: patient preference for regular provider; interpersonal communication with provider; coordination of care; and accumulated knowledge.	-Female provider was significantly associated with perfect ratings for communication and coordination. -Providing gynecologic care was significantly associated with perfect ratings for male and female providers. Patients who used a women's clinic and had a female provider who gave gynecologic care had perfect or nearly perfect ratings for preference for provider, communication, and accumulated knowledge. Gynecologic services are linked to patient ratings of primary care separate from and in synergy with the effect of female provider.
Bean-Mayberry 2003[52]	Female veterans from 8 VA medical centers in 3 states	Females 971	Observational; To compare patient satisfaction in women's clinics (WCs) versus traditional primary care clinics (TCs)	Overall satisfaction and gender-specific satisfaction as measured by the Primary Care Satisfaction Survey for Women (PCSSW)	-Women enrolled in women's clinics were more likely than those in traditional primary care clinics to report excellent overall satisfaction (odds ratio, 1.42; 95% CI, 1.00 to 2.02; p = 0.05). Multivariate models demonstrated that receipt of care in women's clinics was a significant positive predictor for all 5 satisfaction domains (i.e., getting care, privacy and comfort, communication, complete care, and follow-up care) with the gender-specific satisfaction instrument (PCSSW).
Bierman 2007[3]	Male and female veteran VA users with VA pharmacy use	Females 19,115 Males 946,641	Observational; To assess sex differences in rates of inappropriate prescribing before and after accounting for potentially appropriate indications and to examine sex differences in predictors of inappropriate drug use.	Rate of inappropriate prescribing in the elderly by gender using Beers criteria	1)Women were more likely to have received potentially inappropriate medications in all 3 categories: always avoid, rarely appropriate and some indications, even after accounting for diagnosis (always avoid: OR 1.73, 95%CI 1.55-1.94; rarely appropriate: OR 1.18, 95%CI 1.12-1.24; some indications: OR 1.18, 95%CI: 1.14-1.23). 2)In stratified analyses (women only), receiving geriatric care was protective of inappropriate prescribing (OR 0.64, 95%CI 0.53-0.78). 3)Older women in a VA hospital setting are at greater risk for receiving inappropriate drugs than older men.

Author	Sample Characteristics	Sample Size	Design/Objective	Main Measures	Main Findings
Busch 2004[77]	Female and male veteran VA users and non-VA population of employees and retirees with depression diagnosis and initiation of antidepressants.	VA Females 3028 VA Males 24,685 Non-VA Females 3295 Non-VA Males 1557	Observational; To compare quality of pharmacotherapy for patients with major depression in the VA and the private sector.	Quality of depression care pharmacotherapy (HEDIS measure of antidepressant medication management, e.g., proportion of patients with 3 or more follow-up office visits in 12 weeks after depression diagnosis)	1)More than 80% of patients who began anti-depressant treatment achieved guideline-level acute-phase treatment. 2)Few differences in the quality of pharmaco-therapy for depression were found between VA and the private sector, with VA slightly outper-forming in prescription of antidepressants during acute (84.7% vs. 81.0%) and maintenance phases of treatment (53.9% vs. 50.9%). 3)Patient characteristics associated with phar-macotherapy quality included being female, and having a comorbid diagnosis of substance use, bipolar disorder, or anxiety or adjustment disorder.
Chireau 2006[91]	Convenience sample of female veterans who applied for VA maternity benefitsbetween 1999 and 2005	Females 33	Observational; To examine demographic and clinical characteristics of fe-male veterans at the Durham VAMC who were using the VA's fee basis mechanism, their pregnancy outcomes and the costs associated with their pregnancy care	Pregnancy events and outcomes, current medical and psychiatric conditions, and costs	Of the thirty-three veterans with complete records, 61% were white, 39% were black, and mean age was 28.5 years. Ten (32%) had at least one chronic medical condition, and 13 (39%) had at least one psychiatric condition. Adverse pregnancy outcomes occurred in 12 (36%) of the veterans, and most commonly was premature births.
Cypel 2008[80]	National sample of fe-male veterans with active duty orders in Vietnam or other areas between 1967 – 1972	Females 9911	Observational; To compare mortality patterns between Vietnam and non-Vietnam veteran cohorts to the US population	All cause mortality, all cancer mortality, cause specific mortal-ity, crude and adjusted mortality rates, and veteran nurse mortality rates	-Women Vietnam veterans showed a significant deficit (ARR 0.78, 95% CI 0.62, 0.98) in circula-tory system disease relative to non-Vietnam vet-erans, but significant deficits were also observed when both cohorts were compared with women in the U.S. population (SMR 0.65, 95% CI 0.54, 0.77, SMI 0.82, 95% CI 0.73, 0.93, respectively). -Vietnam veterans were at significantly greater risk of mortality from motor vehicle accidents than non-Vietnam veterans (ARE 2.60, 95% CI 1.22, 5.55) and this appeared to be specific to service in Vietnam based upon comparisons to the U.S. population.

Author	Sample Characteristics	Sample Size	Design/Objective	Main Measures	Main Findings
del Junco 2008[85]	Random sample of female patients age 52 years and older from the National Registry of Women Veterans	Females 14093	Observational; To assess internal and external validity in a nationwide, population based trial of an intervention to promote regular mammographic screening	Mammography rates from self report and VHA records for each group of patients	Despite the time lags for baseline survey mailings, respondents in the 5 study groups were similar in race/ethnicity, ever use of VA health care, and age group. Groups 4 and 5 were least likely to respond to the baseline survey or phone calls. At study's end, no between group differences in participant's follow up survey response mode or other characteristics were present. At the year 2 follow up survey, 61% of group 3 reported at least two mammograms since the baseline survey mailing compared to 59% of group 5 (p=.388) in the two years prior to their baseline survey. Overall mammographic coverage was lower in group 5 compared to groups 1-4 combined (82.3% vs. 85.1%, p=.024).
Desai 2005[58]	Female and male VA patient respondents to the National VA Customer Feedback Survey, identified as having a visit to a VA general medicine, primary care, or women's clinic between March 1 - April, 23, 1999, who were not admitted to the hospital in the same time period	Females 5170 Males 45362	Observational; The objective of this study was to assess the role of psychiatric illness in satisfaction with outpatient primary care services in the VA.	core satisfaction with healthcare, including overall coordination of care among providers; open sharing of information with the patient; timeliness and accessibility of service; courtesy of staff; emotional support; coordination of care; specialist provider access; pharmacy access; and continuity of care	After controlling for patient characteristics (e.g., gender, age, disability, acute vs. routine visit) and subjective health, patients with schizophrenia, posttraumatic stress disorder, drug abuse, depression, and other psychiatric disorders reported significantly lower satisfaction with their outpatient primary care. Dissatisfaction was particularly reported for access to care and overall coordination of care.
Etzioni 2006[61]	Female and male VA patients sampled nationally through the VA Office of Quality and Performance (OQP) in fiscal year 2002 (October 1, 2001 to September 30, 2002).	Females 5360 Males 34510	Observational; To examine patterns of colorectal cancer screening and follow-up within the Veterans Health Administration.	Evidence of colorectal cancer screening defined as 1) fecal occult blood test (FOBT; 3 test cards must be returned) in last 12 months, 2) flexible sigmoidoscopy in last 5 years, or 3) colonoscopy in last 10 years; and receipt of follow-up testing after positive FOBT within the follow-up population.	(1) Screening was more likely in patients aged 70 to 80 years than in those younger or older. (2) Female gender, black race, lower income, infrequent primary care visits, and a recent admission to a nursing home were associated with lower likelihood of screening. (3) Forty-one percent of patients were not offered any kind of total colon examination within 6 months of a positive FOBT.

Author	Sample Characteristics	Sample Size	Design/Objective	Main Measures	Main Findings
Fan 2005[57]	Female and male patients in primary care clinics at 7 VA medical centers participating in the Ambulatory Care Quality Improvement Project who returned the baseline Seattle Outpatient Satisfaction Questionnaire (SOSQ) were eligible for this study.	Females 781 Males 20908	Observational; The objective of this trial was to determine whether providing visit-based reports about patient self-reported health status, routine clinical data, and guideline recommendations to providers would improve patient care outcomes	Patient satisfaction with communication skills and humanistic qualities of primary care providers, satisfaction with delivery of health care services, continuity of care (i.e, seeing the same provider), provider characteristics, demographic factors, socioeconomic status, health status, clinic site, patient utilization of services	Increasing self-reported continuity of care was associated with higher patient satisfaction. Patients who reported always seeing the same provider had higher mean humanistic scores and satisfaction scores than those who rarely or never saw the same provider. Female patient gender was associated with improved satisfaction, and increasing age of patient is associated with improved satisfaction until approximately age 70. There was significant variability in mean satisfaction between clinic sites. Patients who received care in primary care clinics within 12 months of returning the questionnaire were more satisfied than those who did not. Among provider characteristics, female clinicians were associated with greater humanistic scores. Provider characteristics were not significantly associated with organizational scores.
Fink 2007[71]	Veteran and non-veteran female surgical patients at VA and private sector hospitals	VA Females 5157 Non-VA Females 27,467	Observational; To test the applicability of the National Surgical Quality Improvement Program (NSQIP) to the private sector in 128 VA hospitals and 14 private academic medical centers for female surgical patients	Unadjusted any cause 30-day mortality inside or outside the hospital, unadjusted morbidity (length of stay, return to the operating room, 19 postoperative complications during the 30-day postop period)	Unadjusted 30-day mortality was virtually identical in the two groups (1.3%). The unadjusted morbidity rate was slightly, but notably, higher in the private sector (10.9%) as compared with that observed in the VA (8.5%, p < 0.0001). The indicator variable for system of care (VA versus private sector) was not statistically significant in the mortality model, but substantially favored the VA in the morbidity model (odds ratio 0.80, 95% CI 0.71, 0.90). Risk-adjusted morbidity is higher in the private sector. The rates of urinary tract infections in the two populations may account for much of the latter difference (3.05% versus 1.75%, p < 0.0001).

Author	Sample Characteristics	Sample Size	Design/Objective	Main Measures	Main Findings
Frayne 2003[79]	National random sample of female veterans using VA ambulatory care	Females 3543	Observational; To determine whether known cardiac risk factors are more prevalent among women veterans who report having sustained sexual assault while in the military	Self-report of current diabetes, hypertension, obesity (BMI ≥ 30), cigarette smoking, problem alcohol use (score > 3 on the TWEAK), sedentary lifestyle (moderate physical activities < 3 times per week), prior hysterectomy (for the subset with age < 40, the premature menopause threshold), and past year cholesterol testing, also current hormone replacement therapy, contact with a medical doctor (in or outside VA) within the past 3 months	-Obesity, smoking, problem alcohol use, sedentary lifestyle, and hysterectomy before age 40 were found to be more common in women reporting a history of sexual assault while in the military than in women without such a history.
Friedemann-Sanchez 2007[66]	Random sample of veterans stratified by sex at Minneapolis VAMC	Females 27 Males 43	Observational; To explore colorectal cancer (CRC) screening barriers, attitudes and preferences by gender.	CRC screening barriers, attitudes, beliefs, preferences, and knowledge and information needs by gender	Female and male participants reported similar preferences for CRC screening mode. Women viewed the preparation for endoscopic procedures as a major barrier to screening while men did not; women and men expressed different fears and information preferences for endoscopic procedures; and women perceive CRC as a male disease thus feeling less vulnerable to it. Pain was foremost issue in the majority of men's minds, and vulnerability in women's.
Haas 2007[32]	All women presenting to the obstetrics clinic for prenatal care appointments at Naval Hospital Camp Lejeune from Jan to Apr 2005	Females 463	Observational; To determine if having a partner deployed in the military during wartime increased the stress levels in pregnant women and to determine predictors of reporting higher stress	Relationship between having a deployed partner and stress levels in pregnant women	Over 88.2% of patients responded to the survey. Women with deployed partners more often reported higher stress levels than those with homeland partners (39.6% and 24.2%, respectively; p<0.01). Logistic regression revealed that having a partner deployed (OR 1.89, 95% CI 1.00-3.57, p=0.04), being active duty (OR 2.64, 95% CI 1.43-4.87, p=<0.01), advanced gestational age (OR 1.04, 95% CI 1.00-1.07, p=0.03) and having >1child at home (OR 2.30, 95% CI 1.12-4.73, p=0.02) all predicted higher stress reporting. Having a support person present was protective against stress (OR 0.40, 95% CI 0.20-0.78, p=<0.01).

Author	Sample Characteristics	Sample Size	Design/Objective	Main Measures	Main Findings
Harriott 2005[56]	Female active duty, stratified random sample of beneficiaries who received maternity care (gave birth) at one of 44 military hospitals between July 1 and September 30, 2001.	Females 2124	Observational; To examine women's evaluations of maternity care with respect to decision-making, confidence, trust in health care providers, and treatment within the military hospital, and to identify aspects of the childbirth experience that were most important to women's recommendations to others of military hospitals.	Patient perceptions of care across multiple dimensions: (1) respect for patient preferences; (2) coordination of care; (3) information and education; (4) attention to physical comfort; (5) emotional support; (6) involvement of family and friends; (7) continuity and transition; and (8) courtesy and availability of staff; overall hospital experience; demographic and clinical information; and assessment of treatment with respect and dignity.	Response Rate was 41%. (1) Less than 50% of respondents would recommend the military hospital to family and friends. (2) The study hospitals had more problems reported than national averages for nearly all dimensions of care. (3) Treatment consistent with individual needs for respect, dignity, and involved decision-making were the primary factors associated with significantly higher overall evaluations; women who expressed higher levels of trust in doctors, midwives, and nurses were more likely to have significantly higher overall evaluations of their care.
Haskell 2004[88]	Female patients identified through VA pharmacy records as taking combination estrogen and progesterone hormone therapy in 1 VA system	Females 48	Observational; To evaluate women's responses to the publication of the Women's Health Initiative (WHI, 2002) and to determine what proportion of women stopped hormone replacement therapy (HRT) and whether the technique of discontinuation affected recurrence of menopausal symptoms.	Cessation of HRT, including abrupt vs. tapered cessation; recurrence of menopausal symptoms.	Over three-quarters (77%) of women stopped taking HRT (20 abruptly and 17 tapered off). Of those women who stopped taking HRT abruptly, 8 (40%) experienced recurrent menopausal symptoms compared to 12 (71%) of those who tapered off of HRT. Tapering off of HRT did not reduce the recurrence of menopausal symptoms compared to abrupt cessation.
Haskell 2007[81]	All female veterans who used VA medical facilities for medical care and also received hormone therapy (HT) through VA pharmacies in 2001	Females 36,222	Observational; To determine whether the decline in HT use nationally also occurred among the population of female veterans taking HT in 2001, and determine if it continued into 2004, and identify whether treatment in a specialized women's health clinic versus other clinics affected HT discontinuation rates	HT medication use was defined as any hormone medication use within the specified calendar year, discontinuation was defined as no longer having any use in the specified year	By 2004, 23,924 (66%) had discontinued HT. Subjects who had used a VA women's clinic or were younger (40-54 years of age) were significantly less likely to discontinue HT. Discontinuation rates in the VA system parallel those in the private sector. However, patients with any use of VA women's clinics were less likely to discontinue HT.

Systematic Review of Women Veterans Health Research 2004-2008

Author	Sample Characteristics	Sample Size	Design/Objective	Main Measures	Main Findings
Hynes 2004[72]	Female and male breast surgery patients with procedures at VA facilities confirmed as having breast cancer using surgical pathology reports were included.	Females 358 Males 120	Observational; To examine trends and outcomes for breast cancer surgery performed at VA hospitals.	30-day morbidity rates (measured as occurrence of 1 or more of 21 complications, such as wound infections, within 30 days), 1-year hospital readmission rates, 30-day mortality, post-operative length of stay (LOS).	1)1,333 breast operations were performed over the course of this 6-year interval (average 1-38/ hospital), with 478 confirmed breast cancer (75% were women). Female breast cancer surgery patients were younger, less likely to be married and more likely to be low income compared to men. Female patients were also more likely to be functionally independent and less likely to have reported frequent alcohol use, to have absent peripheral pulses or to have used steroids. 2)30-day morbidity rates, 1-year hospital readmission rates and 30-day mortality rates were very low for both men and women, post-operative LOS averaged 6.8 days. 3)Lower income, longer operation times and older age increased the likelihood of 30-day morbidity.
Jha 2005[62]	National sample of female and male VA users	6642-86* Females/ Males not specified	Observational;	9 quality measures: 3 preventive services (pneumococcal and influenza vaccinations and colorectal cancer screening); and 6 chronic disease measures (diabetic eye exam screening, annual glycosylated hemoglobin testing [HbA1c], aspirin after myocardial infarction [MI], beta blocker after MI, and blood pressure $\leq$ 140/90 mmHg)	Adjusting for differences in age and hospital characteristics, women and men received comparable care for both preventive care and chronic disease management overall. Age group differences did occur within the quality measures. Among those <65 years, women were more likely to receive HbA1c testing (OR 1.13, 95%CI 1.03-1.25) and adequate hypertension control (OR 1.09, 95%CI 1.00-1.18) but less likely to receive pneumococcal vaccine (OR 0.78, 95%CI 0.73-0.83). While for older patients age >65years, women were less likely to receive adequate hypertension control (OR 0.82, 95%CI 0.75-0.90) and pneumococcal vaccination (OR 0.92, 95% CI 0.86-0.99).

Systematic Review of Women Veterans Health Research 2004-2008

Author	Sample Characteristics	Sample Size	Design/Objective	Main Measures	Main Findings
Johnson 2007[69]	Female patients undergoing vascular surgery at 14 private and 128 VA hospitals	VA Females 458 Non-VA Females 3535	Observational; To compare risk-adjusted 30 day postoperative vascular surgery mortality and morbidity in females in VA and selected University Medical Centers	30 day post-operative morbidity and mortality compared, patient clinical characteristics, and operative data	-Compared with their VA counterparts, women undergoing vascular operations at private sector hospitals had a higher incidence of preoperative co-morbidities; after risk adjustment, mortality did not differ substantially. -Despite risk adjustment, the incidence of postoperative morbidity in the VA patients was considerably lower, suggesting unidentified differences in hospital populations, their processes of care, or both.
Johnson 2006[89]	Female veterans enrolled at the VA Puget Sound Health Care System in 1998	Females 1219	Observational; To determine the prevalence and frequency of mastalgia and its association with psychiatric conditions and unexplained pain syndromes	Breast pain in the past year, categorized as infrequent (1x/month) or frequent (1x/week) mastalgia; posttraumatic stress disorder (PTSD), depression, panic disorder, and alcohol misuse with validated screening tests, self-reported chronic pelvic pain, fibromyalgia, and irritable bowel syndrome	Fifty-five percent of respondents reported past-year mastalgia. Of these, 15% reported frequent mastalgia. Compared to women without mastalgia, women reporting frequent mastalgia were more likely to screen positive for PTSD (OR 5.2, 95% CI 3.2 to 8.4), major depression (OR 4.2, 2.6 to 6.9), panic disorder (OR 7.1, 3.9 to 12.8), eating disorder (OR 2.6, 1.5 to 4.7), alcohol misuse (OR 1.8, 1.1 to 2.8), or domestic violence (OR 3.1, 1.9 to 5.0), and to report fibromyalgia (OR 3.9, 2.1 to 7.4), chronic pelvic pain (OR 5.4, 2.7 to 10.5), or irritable bowel syndrome (OR 2.8, 1.6 to 4.8).
Johnson 2006[78]	All female veteran VA users in local area of 1 VA Healthcare System	Females 1555	Observational; To describe the association between obesity and television viewing practices among women veterans.	Presence of overweight or obesity by body mass index, television viewing practices, physical activity, screening for depression and PTSD	-Watching television >2 hours per day and eating or snacking while watching television were each associated with obesity (OR 1.4, 95% CI 1.1, 1.8; and OR 1.3, 95% CI 1.0, 1.7, respectively), after adjusting for patient characteristics. Results were similar when PTSD was included in model instead of depression. -Women who both watched >2 hours of television per day and ate or snacked while viewing were almost twice as likely to be obese (OR 1.9, 95% CI 1.4, 2.6).

Author	Sample Characteristics	Sample Size	Design/Objective	Main Measures	Main Findings
Katzburg 2009[65]	Female veteran smokers	Females 33	Observational/Qualitative; To design a new smoking cessation program tailored for women veterans	Identify critical components of an ideal smoking cessation program	Women veterans identified critical components of an ideal program, emotional support and choice, suggesting the need for a personalized program. The Expert Panel designed an individualized menu-driven smoking cessation program that included five programs as well as a variety of quit/support tools. In the pilot, women completing the designed booklet selected multiple menu options, demonstrating enthusiasm for program components. The traditional VA program was the least selected program option.
Katzburg 2008[64]	Female veteran smokers with a visit at one of the two VA Greater Los Angeles women's clinics in the past year	Females 23	Observational/Qualitative; To report on the results of 4 focus groups with female smokers emphasizing the components of an ideal program to identify potential new smoking cessation interventions.	Descriptive themes for an ideal smoking cessation group for women	Support and choice were the major themes culled from the descriptive analyses. Types of support included educational and emotional support from professional, peer and self-support mechanisms. Informal and formal peer-support mechanisms were supported in the form of a buddy/sponsor or traditional alcoholics anonymous program style. Choice was a theme repeated across groups in discussions of choices of support, formats for support (individual face to face, telephone, email), or the tangible components of a program.
Korthius 2004[63]	Female and male veterans with HIV infection treated at VA facilities	Females 59 Males 4006	Observational; To assess the level of adherence to lipid screening guidelines among providers caring for HIV-infected veterans exposed to protease inhibitors (PI) and to identify facility-level predictors of adherence to lipid-screening guidelines.	lipid screening within first 6 months of PI use; number of months from first PI use to triglyceride/lipid test	(1)Six in 10 veterans taking PIs received recommended lipid screening. (2)In the full model, older age, Latino ethnicity, diabetes, hyperlipidemia history, and urban location are positive predictors of lipid screening, while IVDU exposure, heterosexual orientation, and unknown HIV risk were negative predictors of lipid screening by 6 months.

Author	Sample Characteristics	Sample Size	Design/Objective	Main Measures	Main Findings
Lang 2005[55]	Female veterans who utilized the VA San Diego Healthcare System in 1998 at five different sites	Females 221	Observational; To examine the association between satisfaction with general medical services and trauma-related mental health symptoms in women.	overall satisfaction with visit; satisfaction with the provider; satisfaction with the clinic	The majority of patients were pleased with care they received. Older age and better mental health were significantly associated with greater overall satisfaction. The association between PTSD symptoms and satisfaction approached significance. Only general mental health reached significance individually with both satisfaction with the provider and the clinic. Women with more PTSD symptoms appear to be more satisfied with their overall care and with their provider.
Lautz 2007[70]	Female and male VA and non-VA (private sector, PS) gastric bypass surgery patients from 12 VA medical centers and 12 private sector medical centers	VA Female 112; VA Male 262; Non-VA Female 1656; Non-VA Male 408	Observational; To evaluate outcomes and predictors of morbidity in VA and non-VA (PS) patients undergoing Roux-en-Y gastric bypass (RYGB) during the Patient Safety in Surgery (PSS) Study	patient demographics (age, race), preoperative co-morbidities (smoking, alcohol use, history of co-morbid conditions, pulmonary and central nervous system function), preoperative laboratory values, and variables related to the operation (hospital type, open surgical procedure), and 30-day post surgical outcomes	-The odds of postoperative morbidity for VA versus PS female patients was 1.14 (95% CI, 0.63-2.05), and for male patients 2.29 (95% CI, 1.28-4.10). -The VA male subset showed higher risk-adjusted postoperative morbidity compared with the PS male subset. The VA and PS female subsets had equivalent risk-adjusted post-operative morbidity.
Maciejewski 2005[97]	Female and male veterans (from a prior study trial) with a primary care provider and at least one primary care visit in the year prior to the study intervention	Females 217 Males 14232	Observational; To evaluate the performance of different prospective risk adjustment models of outpatient, inpatient, and total expenditures of veterans who regularly use Veterans Affairs (VA) primary care	Total expenditures of VA care during a 1-year period from the index date based on the sum of inpatient and outpatient expenditures.	In all expenditure models, administrative-based measures performed better than self-reported measures, which performed better than age and gender. Prior outpatient expenditures predicted outpatient expenditures best by far (R^2=42 percent). Models with multiple measures improved overall prediction, reduced over-prediction of low expenditure quintiles, and reduced under-prediction in the highest quintile of expenditures.
Maguen 2005[83]	Transgender (male to female) veterans who consented to participate in one VA facility	Females 6	Observational/Qualitative; To provide a case study description of a cognitive behavioral therapy (CBT) program for transgender male to female (MTF) veterans	Demographic data, qualitative illustrations	Most participants (n=4) experienced the following issues: employment problems; housing issues; lack of social support; anxiety or depression; significant trauma history; and PTSD symptoms. Women in the group showed improvement on measures of anxiety and depression from pre- to post-treatment. The group appeared to reduce transgender related isolation and stigma.

Systematic Review of Women Veterans Health Research 2004-2008

Author	Sample Characteristics	Sample Size	Design/Objective	Main Measures	Main Findings
McEachrane-Gross 2006[96]	Female and male veterans using the outpatient oncology or pain clinics at the Jamaica Plains campus of the Boston Healthcare System	Females 17 Males 245	Observational; To measure the prevalence of selected complementary and alternative medicine (CAM) use among veterans attending oncology and chronic pain clinics, and to describe the characteristics of CAM use in this population	Use of 6 common CAM (herbs, dietary supplements, chiropractic care, massage therapy, acupuncture and homeopathy)	Seventy-two patients (27.3%) reported CAM use within the past 12 months. CAM use was associated with more education (p = 0.02), higher income (p = 0.006), non-VA insurance (p = 0.003), additional care outside the VA (p = 0.01) and the belief that lifestyle contributes to illness (p = 0.015). The diagnosis of chronic pain versus cancer was not associated with differential CAM use (p = 0.15). No difference in CAM use occurred by gender; however, women were only 7% of the sample.
McQueen 2008[98]	National sample of women veterans aged 52 years or older who were participating in a repeat mammography intervention trial	Females 3414	Observational; To examine predictors or three single-item measures of patient perceived susceptibility to breast cancer (absolute perceived risk, ordinal risk, and comparative risk likelihood (i.e., their own risk compared with other women)	Perceived risk, demographics, health status, health behaviors	Breast symptoms and greater cancer worry increased patient perceived susceptibility to breast cancer for all 3 dependent measures. Other predictors varied by dependent measure.
Miller 2008[92]			Observational; To assess incidence of angioedema and the potential determinants.	Angioedema cases among patients on antihypertensives; angioedema rates by angiotensin converting enzyme inhibitors (ACE) or other antihypertensive agents; relative risk for angioedema by ACE or other agent	Overall, 0.20% of ACE initiators developed angioedema while on the medication and incidence rate was 1.97 cases per 1000 person years. The rate of angioedema on other agents initiated was 0.51, and the adjusted relative risk estimate was 3.56 (2.82-4.44). 55% of cases occurred within 90 days of first ACE use. Nearly 58.3% of angioedema cases were estimated to be due to starting ACE. Angioedema rates were 50% higher in women. However, no female specific incidence data were presented.

Author	Sample Characteristics	Sample Size	Design/Objective	Main Measures	Main Findings
Mrus 2006[95]	Convenience sample of veterans and nonveterans presenting at either a VA medical center or a non-VA medical center (4 sites)	Females 63 Males 387	Observational; To compare health-related quality of life (HRQoL) between patients receiving care in Veterans Administration (VA) settings (veterans) and non-VA settings (non-veterans), and to explore determinants of HRQoL and change in HRQoL over time in subjects living with HIV/AIDS	Determinants of HRQoL which included health status, health ratings, etc (e.g., overall function, symptom bother, health ratings)	Compared with nonveterans, the veteran population was older and consisted of a higher proportion of males. On scales ranging from 0 (worst) to 100 (best), veterans reported significantly poorer overall function. Determinants associated with multiple HRQoL outcomes in multivariable analyses were: symptom bother, overall function, religiosity/spirituality, depressive symptoms, and financial worries. Only 14% of the overall sample was female and differed by veteran status. Increased number of bothersome symptoms was associated with female gender.
Pierce 1999[42]	Stratified, random sample of US Air Force military women selected from a Department of Defense database who served in Operation Desert Shield or Desert Storm	Females 525	Observational; To provide baseline health information on a randomized sample of military women serving during the Persian Gulf War.	Prevalence of gender specific health problems, rate of health care utilization, satisfaction with military and civilian care during respondents' military careers	-The most prevalent gender-specific problems were problems during pregnancy (41%), urinary tract infection (34%), headache (33%), and menstrual irregularities (32%) and abnormal Pap smear (27%). - Of note, many women did not seek health care for their problems. -In this overall group, 76% reported using military health care, 41% used civilian health care, and only 3% reported using the VA for care. -Overall, for 15 of 18 conditions, satisfaction ratings were higher for civilian care.

Author	Sample Characteristics	Sample Size	Design/Objective	Main Measures	Main Findings
Pugh 2006[74]	Male and female veteran VA users with VA pharmacy use	Females 21,342 Males 1,075,019	Observational; To use HEDIS 2006 criteria to determine the rate of potentially inappropriate prescribing in the elderly (PIPE) and to determine if patient risk factors are similar to those found using Beers criteria.	Rate of inappropriate prescribing in the elderly using HEDIS 2006 criteria	1) Results for the HEDIS 2006 measure were similar to those of the 1997 Beers criteria. 2) Overall, 19.6% of the cohort received at least 1 drug included in the HEDIS 2006 criteria, and 3.9% received 2 or more HEDIS 2006 drugs; the oldest of the elderly were at lower risk of PIPE and the youngest of the elderly were at greater risk. 3) Rates of PIPE varied between women and men (23.3% of women and 19.2% of men received 1 or more HEDIS drugs). 4) The count of unique drugs was the strongest predictor for both men and women: the risk increased for those receiving 10 or more drugs (men adjusted OR 8.2, 95%CI 8.0-8.4; women adjusted OR 9.6, 95%CI 8.2-11.2).
Pugh 2005[76]	Female and male veterans aged 65 and older having at least one VA outpatient visit in Fiscal Year 2000	VA Females 25,309 VA Males 1,240,125	Observational; To identify inappropriate prescribing using criteria for proper use developed by the Agency for Healthcare Research and Quality and dose-limitation criteria defined by Beers, and to describe duration of use and patient characteristics associated with inappropriate prescribing for older adults	Appropriate use/inappropriate use of drugs; patient characteristics and duration of use associated with inappropriate use	After adjusting for diagnoses, dose, and duration, inappropriate prescribing decreased from 33% to 23% and exposure to inappropriate drugs was prolonged. Pain relievers, benzodiazepines, antidepressants, and musculoskeletal agents constituted 61% of inappropriate prescribing. Whites, patients with psychiatric comorbidities, and patients receiving more medications were mostly likely to receive inappropriate drugs. Women were more likely to receive Zhan criteria drugs; men were more likely to receive dose-limited drugs.

Author	Sample Characteristics	Sample Size	Design/Objective	Main Measures	Main Findings
Sohn 2006[87]	All female and male VHA users 18 years or older who were veterans and used either inpatient or outpatient care in the VA in the current or previous year		Observational; To describe the prevalence rates of urologic cancers and selected benign urologic conditions and their trends between 1999 and 2002 for those who have been using healthcare from the VA	Prevalence rates of 8 high priority urologic diseases including prostate, bladder, and kidney cancers, renal mass, interstitial cystitis, prostatitis, erectile dysfunction, and urethral stricture, and 13 overall urologic conditions (also includes peyronies disease, infertility, undescended testis, hypospadias, and testicular cancer).	Among conditions evaluated, prostate cancer was listed as a primary diagnosis for 5.4% of VHA users in 2002, followed in decreasing prevalence by erectile dysfunction (2.9%), renal mass (1.5%), interstitial cystitis (14%), and prostatitis (1.1%). Age-adjusted rates showed significant increases for renal mass (31%), interstitial cystitis (14%), and erectile dysfunction (8%) between 1999 and 2002. While no major findings are reported by gender, interstitial cystitis was almost twice as prevalent among female compared to male users.
Straits-Troster 2006[67]	Female and male random sample of veterans receiving care at VA outpatient clinics during the November 2003 – March 2004 influenza season	Females 4053 Males 113561	Observational; To assess racial/ethnic differences in influenza vaccination in VA and to examine barriers to and facilitators of influenza vaccination among veteran outpatients aged 50 years and older.	Influenza vaccination barriers and facilitators	In the multivariate model used to calculate adjusted prevalence, age accounted for most of the racial/ethnic differences, although non-Hispanic blacks were still significantly less likely to report influenza vaccination compared to non-Hispanic whites. Gender did not have an effect on vaccination in the univariate or multivariate model. Reminder by a member of the patient's VA healthcare team was the most frequently endorsed factor for vaccination (42.4%), followed by facility poster displays (20.8%), and family or friend's reminder to get a vaccination (12.7%).
Tseng 2006[59]	Female and male veterans with diabetes who used VA care, were age 65+, and enrolled in Medicare	Females 3225 Males 231,922	Observational; To examine gender differences in diabetes care process measures and intermediate outcomes among veteran clinic users	Diabetes process of care measures included: hemoglobin A1c (HbA1c); low density lipoprotein cholesterol (LDL-C); and eye exams. Intermediate outcomes included HbA1c and LDL-C values.	Overall, there were no significant gender differences in HbA1c or LDL-C testing. However, women had higher rates of these process measures than men among the non-African American minorities. Women were more likely to have completed eye exams (OR 1.11, 99% CI 1.10, 1.23) but were less likely to have LDL-C under 130mg/dL (OR 0.77, 99% CI 0.69, 0.87).

Author	Sample Characteristics	Sample Size	Design/Objective	Main Measures	Main Findings
Tseng 2006[60]	Female veteran VA users with diabetes and disability, under age 65, and alive at the end of FY 2000	Females 2344	Observational; To analyze predictors of diabetes care consistent with performance standards among women VA clinic users with disability enrollment status (i.e., service connection)	Process measures included ≥ 1 test for glycosylated hemoglobin (HbA1c), low density lipoprotein cholesterol (LDL-C), and an eye examination in FY 2000, and intermediate outcomes included HbA1c levels and LCL-C levels for VA data only.	(1) Veteran women with disability were more likely to receive recommended tests compared to veteran women without disability. (2) Women with disability were more likely to have poor LDL-C control than men with disability; women with disability were more likely to have LDL-C testing and less likely to have poor HbA1c control compared to men with disability. (3) There is a lack of demographic, socioeconomic, and health status predictors on HbA1c control and LDL-C control, except for the association between the African-American race and poor HbA1c control. (4) Among women with disability, older veteran women were more likely to be tested for HbA1c and LDL-C values.
Vander Weg 2008[68]	Female and male active duty recruits who entered Air Force Basic Military Training during the period from October 1999 to September 2000.	Females 7826 Males 23281	Observational; To evaluate the use of several different alternative tobacco products (bidis, cigars, kreteks, pipes, and smokeless tobacco [ST]) in a large sample of young adults who are vulnerable to tobacco use given their age and military status.	Four general domains were assessed, including demographics, tobacco use history, potential risk factors for tobacco use, and other health risk behaviors.	Use of any type of alternative tobacco product was significantly greater among cigarette smokers compared to non-cigarette smokers. Use of alternative tobacco products was consistently higher for males than for females. The one exception was kreteks, where prevalence rates did not differ by gender.
Vernon 2008[9]	Random sample of female veterans 52years and older from the National Registry of Women Veterans	Females 2681	Experimental; To evaluate strategies to increase regular mammography screening, compare rates of completion of two or more mammograms among women randomly assigned to a tailored and targeted intervention, only targeted intervention, or survey-only control group	Self-reported mammography coverage (completion of one postintervention mammogram) and compliance (completion of two postintervention mammograms)	In none of the primary analyses did the tailored and targeted intervention result in higher mammography rates than the targeted-only intervention, and there was limited support for either intervention being more effective than the baseline survey alone.

Author	Sample Characteristics	Sample Size	Design/Objective	Main Measures	Main Findings
Vogt 2008[8]	Male and female VA employees who have patient contact at 2 VA sites	Females 89 Males 69	Randomized Educational Trial To evaluate random assignment to educational intervention versus control group. (2 group, pretest/posttest)	Evaluation of gender-role ideology, knowledge and sensitivity among VA employees	-Older age, direct patient contact, and years of VA employment predicted higher gender awareness and suggests a meaningful role for 'hands-on' experience. -Analyses revealed significantly greater improvement in sensitivity and knowledge for participants in intervention relative to control setting. -Contrary to expectations, the program did not result in significant improvements in gender-role ideology.
von Sadovszky 2007[86]	Female Army personnel recruited from Army posts or reserve units throughout the U.S.	Females 131	Observational; To ascertain Army women's specific sexual health information needs prior to developing a theoretically based, self-administered intervention to promote safer sexual practices during deployment.	Descriptive statistics for sexual risk variables, types of information received in the past and from whom, whether or not more information was desired	Participants had moderate levels of sexual risk behaviors. Forced-choice responses yielded little desire for information regarding safer sexual practices. Women identified different sexual health and safer sexual information needs based upon whether they were at a normal duty station or during deployment.
Washington 2007[51]	VA-eligible female veterans from one city, who were VA users and non-users	Females 51	Observational; To determine women veterans' perspectives and decision-making about VA health care use	Information needs, access, gender appropriateness of services and gender-related aspects of care, quality of care	-Barriers to VA use for both VA users and nonusers included lack of information about eligibility and available services. -Nonusers often assumed the VA did not provide women's health care. -All groups emphasized a requirement for a health care system focused on quality and sensitivity to women's health issues. However, users and nonusers differed in perceptions of VA quality. -VA environment and quality concerns led many women to limit their VA use to women's clinics.

Systematic Review of Women Veterans Health Research 2004-2008

Author	Sample Characteristics	Sample Size	Design/Objective	Main Measures	Main Findings
Weeks 2006[94]	National sample of veterans the 1999 Large Health Survey of Veteran Enrollees who used VA for care and had at least 1 of 30 physical health diagnoses	Females 23984 Males 546528	Observational; To determine whether urban/ rural disparities persist when examining disease categories of rural and urban methods.	Health related quality of life scores (HRQoL) using the SF-36 physical component score and mental component score (PCS and MCS); 30 physical disease diagnoses (ICD-9-CM)	Most diseases were significantly more prevalent in the rural veteran population. In adjusted and unadjusted analyses, PCS was significantly lower for veterans in rural settings, and MCS was lower, but differences were less pronounced. In the multivariate adjusted regression model, female gender was significantly associated with mean PCS and MCS scores (gender difference in PCS: Coefficient: 0.47, $p<0.0001$; gender difference in MCS: Coefficient: 2.33, $p<0.0001$).
Wright 2006[53]	Female and male VA outpatients and inpatients who responded to a mailed Survey of Healthcare Experiences of Patients (SHEP) in fiscal year 2004.	Female 5244 Males 128,318	Observational; To compare patient satisfaction of male and female users of Veterans Health Administration (VA) services.	Patient ratings of overall quality and unique dimensions of satisfaction; socio-demographic and health related patient characteristics	In adjusted analyses, overall quality and most dimensions of satisfaction were not different for females compared to males. However, continuity of care was rated higher by females in outpatient care. Additionally, for inpatient quality, men reported higher scores after adjustment for transitions (68 vs. 65, $p=0.0009$), physical comfort (82 vs. 80, $p=0.0003$), involvement of family and friends (74 vs. 71, $p=0.0024$), courtesy (88 vs. 86, $p=0.0001$), coordination (77 vs. 74, $p=0.0000$), and access (80 vs. 76, $p=0.0000$). Women were less satisfied than men in inpatient settings. Women may be more aware of being a minority in a hospital than in outpatient settings.
Yu 2006[93]	Final nursing home stays of all patients (n=4,879) who died in VA nursing homes between October 1, 1999, and September 30, 2000 and were 65 years or older at death	Females 117 Males 4762	Observational; To examine the final stays of elderly patients (65 and older) who died in 111 VA nursing homes in fiscal year 2000 and to evaluate the determinants of costs of final nursing home stays.	Primary outcome measure is cost; also analyzed length of stay (LOS) and intensity of care to understand how cost is associated with these study factors.	Patients with service-related conditions had higher costs, longer LOS, and similar RUG scores in all three models. Having a living spouse was not significant in the demographic-only model for cost and LOS but was strongly significant when controlling for medical conditions for other models (2 and 3). Overall, all of the independent variables appear to be affecting costs through LOS alone, with the exception of having a living spouse and stroke. Gender was not a significant factor for cost of LOS in the generalized linear regressions.

APPENDIX 8. ACCESS AND UTILIZATION EVIDENCE TABLE

Author	Sample Characteristics	Sample Size	Design/Objective	Main Measures	Main Findings
Bean-Mayberry 2008[100]	Random sample of female veterans in 10 regional VAMCs, with an outpatient visit in primary care or women's clinic between 3/1/1999 – 3/1/2000	Females 1051	Observational; To compare female veterans who use the VA for primary care with female veterans who use both VA and non-VA providers (dual use) and identify the health care factors associated with dual use	Dual use of VA and non-VA providers	Having a VA provider perform general gynecologic care (OR 0.37, 95%CI 0.22, 0.60) and use of a VA women's clinic (OR 0.56, 95%CI 0.35, 0.90) were each associated with significantly lower odds of dual use. Dissatisfaction with overall VA care (OR 1.88, 95%CI 1.04, 3.41) and higher income (OR 1.89, 95%CI 1.32, 2.71) were significantly associated with higher odds of dual use. Female provider had no effect on dual use (OR 0.87, 95%CI 0.53, 1.40).
Borrero 2006[117]	Female and male VA patients in fiscal year 1999, age 50 years or older with or without the diagnosis of osteoarthritis (OA) in any joint were included.	Females 44569 Males 1,923,524	Observational; To examine gender differences in the utilization rates of total knee/hip arthroplasty in the Veterans Administration (VA) system.	Primary outcome was undergoing knee or hip total joint arthroplasty within 2 years (fiscal years 2000 and 2001).	Of the total 1,968,093 (2.3% women) VA patients in FY 1999 who were 50 years of age or older, 329,461 (2.9% women) patients carried a diagnosis of OA. For women, the 2-year adjusted odds of undergoing total knee or hip arthroplasty was 0.97 (95%CI 0.83 to 1.14) and 1.00 (95%CI 0.79 to 1.27), respectively yielding no statistically significant gender differences within the study period.
Carney 2003[141]	Female and male population based sample in the Iowa Gulf War Study who were on active duty/ activated and deployed in the Persian Gulf War between August 1990 and July 1991.	Females 129 Males 1767	Observational; To provide a descriptive study of women and men who were deployed to the region of the Gulf War in order to compare their combat experiences, occupational exposures, and self reported use of health care services 5 years after deployment.	Environmental and combat exposures, health care utilization	No significant deployment differences were seen by gender; lengths of stay, locations deployed, and primary occupation groups were similar by gender. Similar overall mean numbers of combat and noncombat exposures were experienced by women and men(10 ± 0.4 vs. 10 ± 0.1). Men reported a higher level of preparedness for combat and more frequently participated in combat. Compared to men, women were more likely to have more than 5 outpatient visits during the previous year, have an inpatient hospitalization, and receive VA compensation.

Author	Sample Characteristics	Sample Size	Design/Objective	Main Measures	Main Findings
Chen 2007[120]	National sample of homeless veterans who had an outreach intake and first contact with the Health Care for Homeless Veterans (HCHV) program at any of the VAMC sites	Females 188 Males 5543	Observational; To identify factors associated with receipt of VA pension and compensation benefits among homeless veterans after their initial contact with the VA national homeless (community) outreach program.	Proportion of homeless veterans who were awarded any benefits; sociodemographic, clinical, and military service characteristics of beneficiaries and nonbeneficiaries in the program and those who receive pension benefits or compensation benefits	Female veterans were more likely to receive compensation benefits than pension benefits. Homeless female veterans might be less likely than male veterans to be referred to VA mental health services by non-VA clinicians because clinicians might not ask whether the women were veterans. A limited number of veterans (15%) were subsequently awarded benefits; they were more likely to have reported recent use of VA services and a greater number of medical and psychiatric problems at the time of outreach.
Dobie 2006[29]	Female veterans receiving care between 10/01/1996 - 1/01/2000 at VA Puget Sound Health Care System	Females 2578	Observational; To determine associations between medical/surgical utilization and PTSD in female patients	Rates of medical/surgical hospitalizations, surgical inpatient procedures, and outpatient utilization for PTSD positive and PTSD negative women.	Female veterans who screen positive for PTSD receive more VA medical/surgical services. About 33% of the women screened positive for PTSD. PTSD+ women had higher rates of medical/surgical hospitalizations of 20% vs. 14% overall. In particular, PTSD+ women ages 35-49 had significantly more mean hospital days compared to PTSD- women (43 vs. 17 days, $p<.0001$). Similarly, more PTSD+ women ages 35-49 underwent surgical procedures (5.9% vs. 1.7%, $p<.001$). Mean annual outpatient visits were also significantly higher among PTSD+ women ($p<.001$ for each comparison).
Erbes 2007[15]	Female and male OEF/OIF veteran enrollees at one Midwestern VAMC who had returned within a six-month time frame	Females 17 Males 103	Observational; To evaluate levels of PTSD, depression, alcohol abuse, quality of life, and mental health service utilization among returnees from Operation Enduring Freedom and Operation Iraqi Freedom (OEF/OIF).	psychiatric distress levels (PTSD symptoms using PCL, depression using Beck Depression scale, and alcohol use using AUDIT), functional impairment, and service utilization	PTSD levels (12%) were consistent with previous research while problematic drinking levels were also elevated (33%). PTSD and, to a lesser degree, alcohol abuse were associated with lower quality of life in multiple domains, even when controlling for the influence of depression. Of those screening positive for PTSD, 56% reported using mental health services. Only 18% of those screening positive for alcohol abuse reported using such services. No reported findings related to gender.

Systematic Review of Women Veterans Health Research 2004-2008

Author	Sample Characteristics	Sample Size	Design/Objective	Main Measures	Main Findings
Fontana 2006[135]	Female veterans with consecutive admissions to the Women's Stress Disorder Treatment Team (WSDTT) at 4 VA sites.	Females 224	Observational; To examine the role of women's comfort in coming for treatment of PTSD in a predominantly male environment	Female veterans comfort level when entering treatment and while participating in therapy, socio-demographic and clinical characteristics associated with comfort level, and strength of association of comfort level and participation and satisfaction with treatment.	(1) As a group, women treated for military-related stress disorder were "somewhat comfortable" in coming to the VA for specialized PTSD treatment from the start. The most important factor contributing to their level of comfort was the availability of a specialized treatment program for women. (2) Women who had prior contact with the VA reported no change in comfort level over the 8-month period. Women who did not have prior contact with the VA reported an increase in comfort from intake to 4 months. (3) Among women who did not have prior contact with the VA, those of minority ethnicity had significantly lower comfort levels, and, among women who did have prior contact with the VA, those with higher levels of education had significantly lower comfort levels. (4) Among women, comfort level did not have a significant effect on their satisfaction with treatment.
Frayne 2008[112]	National sample of all female and male (veteran and non-veterans) in FY2002 VA enrollee database	Female veterans 178,849 Male veterans 3,943,532 Female Non-vets 183,722; Male Non-vets 123,311	Observational; To determine whether gender differences in VA utilization and cost change when comparing all VA users versus the veteran only cohort.	Total # outpatient encounters in FY 2002; primary care visits in FY 2002; inpatient length of stay; cost of outpatient care and inpatient care	-Nonveterans accounted for 50.7% of women (the majority employees) but only 3.0% of men. -Among all VA users, women were younger and less likely to have a medical or mental health condition. -However, veteran women were more likely to have a mental health condition than veteran men, and more likely to have 3 or more primary care visits during the year. Women veterans had a higher mean # of visits compared to men veterans and a higher cost for outpatient care (p<.001). Women veterans also had lower inpatient utilization and cost (p<.001).

Author	Sample Characteristics	Sample Size	Design/Objective	Main Measures	Main Findings
Frayne 2006[111]	Female and male veterans in VA administrative databases in FY 2002 (outpatient, inpatient, pharmacy); non-veterans are excluded	Female veterans 178849; Male veterans 3,943,532;	Observational; To examine how utilization and cost of VHA care differ between female and male veterans	Number of inpatient days and outpatient encounters; costs of inpatient, outpatient and pharmacy care	-Women had 10.9% fewer inpatient encounters, 1.3% more outpatient encounters, and significantly lower total costs (-2.8%) and lower inpatient costs (-20.8%) compared to men (p<.001 for each comparison). -Women veterans utilized more outpatient services if they had both medical and mental health conditions compared to men. -Women veterans were significantly younger, unmarried, more often service connected, and more often had mental health diagnoses.
Frueh 2007[131]	Random sample of female and male veterans less than 80 years old at 4 VAMC primary care clinics selected in fiscal year 1999	Females 50 Males 695	Observational; To expand our understanding of PTSD prevalence, its psychiatric characteristics, and service use among elderly veterans in VA primary care clinics	prevalence of PTSD and psychiatric diagnoses by age; physical and mental health functioning by age; use of VA mental health services and disability benefits; identification of explanatory characteristics	Those in the 45–64 year age group endorsed the highest scores and those in the oldest age group (65 and older) endorsed the lowest scores, even after adjusting for the effects of race and sex. Similarly, those in the oldest group (7.5%) had one-third of the prevalence of major depression as those in the two younger groups (21.7% and 22.9%), and they had a lower prevalence of other psychiatric conditions, such as panic disorder, agoraphobia, social anxiety, and substance abuse. They also were about half as likely to show evidence of suicidal risk. In all cases, these differences were maintained even after controlling for relevant demographic covariates, such as race and sex. Those in the 45–64 year old group were generally more likely to meet criteria for most psychiatric disorders, followed by the 18–44 group, and then the 65 and older group. All but one of these relationships remained significant after adjusting for the effects of race and sex. The one exception was in rates of substance abuse/dependence between the 45–64 and 65 and older groups.

Author	Sample Characteristics	Sample Size	Design/Objective	Main Measures	Main Findings
Greenberg 2004[137]	Female veterans entering outpatient treatment for PTSD at one of 4 VA Women's Stress Disorders Treatment Programs (Boston, Brecksville, Loma Linda, New Orleans).	Females 149	Observational; To examine the strength of association between continuity of care and health outcomes for female veterans newly entering outpatient treatment for PTSD.	Changes in clinical status between program entry and four months follow-up on 11 measures (e.g., PTSD symptoms, general psychiatric/physical health, alcohol and drug abuse, violent behavior).	1) Few significant associations between continuity and outcomes were found. 2) Four months after program entry, only commitment to treatment (treatment process) was positively associated with one or more continuity of care measures. 3) Severity continuity of care measures were associated with poor health outcomes. 4) Eight months after program entry, patients with greater continuity of care during the first four months of treatment had greater declines in violent behavior and PTSD measurements and larger increases in global functioning. 5) However, corrections for multiple comparison resulted in no statistically significant relationships, demonstrating only weak and inconsistent evidence of the clinical benefits of continuity of care for women entering care for PTSD.
Grubaugh 2006[130]	Randomly identified female veterans who attended primary care clinic in any of the four VA sites in fiscal year 1999 (Charleston and Columbia, SC; Tuscaloosa and Birmingham, AL)	Females 187	Observational; To examine rates of medical and psychiatric disorders among female veterans, the recognition of such disorders by VAMC care providers, and the use of relevant medical and mental health services by women both within and outside of the VA setting	Frequency of psychiatric diagnoses, diagnostic accuracy, and medical comorbidity; Frequency of medical disorders and medical and psychiatric comorbidity; Functioning (SF-36 mental & physical health composite scores); Use of VA Health Services by psychiatric diagnosis; Use of outside care	Forty-four percent (43.9%) of women met criteria for at least one psychiatric disorder; 34.0% of these women met criteria for two or more additional psychiatric diagnoses, and concordance rates between interview and chart diagnoses were low. Ninety-five percent (95.2%) of women had a medical condition noted in their charts; 86.6% had two or more additional medical conditions, and a significant number of women had both medical and psychiatric diagnoses. Forty-four percent (43.9%) of women with an identified mental health condition received specialized mental health care by the VA in the past year.

Author	Sample Characteristics	Sample Size	Design/Objective	Main Measures	Main Findings
Haskell 2008[81]	National Sample of women VA users identified through pharmacy benefits data in 2001 as receiving a prescription for oral conjugated equine estrogen, estradiol, the estradiol patch or any estrogen preparation in combination with medroxyprogesterone as hormone therapy (HT)	Females 36,222	Observational; To (1) determine whether the decline in HT use nationally also occurred among female veterans taking HT in 2001, occurred after 2002 during 2003 and 2004, and (2) determine whether treatment in a specialized women's health clinic versus other clinic settings affected HT discontinuation rates.	Any HT use within the specified calendar year, regardless of duration of use; discontinuation was defined as no longer having any use in the specified year.	In 2001, 36,222 female veterans used HT. By 2004, 23,924 (66%) had discontinued HT. Subjects who used a VA women's clinic or were younger (40-54 years of age) were significantly less likely to discontinue HT. However, Hispanic panic ethnicity, African American race, and clinical diagnoses such as heart disease and mastectomy were significantly associated with discontinuation. Discontinuation rates in the VA parallel those in the private sector. However, patients with any use of VA women's clinics were less likely to discontinue HT, indicating a practice setting variation that may indicate either more specific care or differential implementation of the new HT guidelines.
Haskell 2006[121]	Convenience sample of women veterans receiving care in the VA Connecticut Women's Health Center	Females 213	Observational; To provide descriptive data about pain among women veterans receiving care in a VA primary care setting	Prevalence of pain and key pain dimensions in a sample of women veterans	(1) Most women veterans (78%) reported an ongoing pain problem with a mean duration of 6 years, average pain intensity of 6.3 (range 1-10), and most commonly endorsed pain sites included lower extremity (68%), low back (63%), and shoulder (48%). (2) Women older than 65 years reported lower use of pain treatments. (3) Those with pain (vs. without) were more than 6 times as likely to report ≥12 medical visits in the past year and twice as likely to report ≥12 visits to a mental health provider.

Author	Sample Characteristics	Sample Size	Design/Objective	Main Measures	Main Findings
Hatmaker 2006[116]	Female patients who presented to VA General Surgery Clinic at one site with a breast mass or abnormal mammogram from 2003 to 2005.	Females 62	Observational; To examine the costs and trends in the use of surgical versus percutaneous image-guided biopsy procedures.	Number and type of procedures each year, location of procedure (VA or non-VA hospital) and total costs associated with open or percutaneous biopsies were calculated.	(1) The average total cost to evaluate a patient with a breast mass or mammographic abnormality through an open biopsy in the operating room at the VA hospital was $4,368 (SD, $2,586) with a median cost of $3,479. (2) The average total cost for a percutaneous image-guided breast biopsy was $1,267 (SD, $536) with a median cost of $1,239. (3) A 3.8-fold increase in the use of percutaneous image-guided techniques for the evaluation of breast lesions over a recent 3-year period was observed. (4) For VA with available resources, the option of image-guided percutaneous biopsy techniques is a cost-effective and more preferable alternative to open surgical biopsy.
Hoge 2006[20]	Female and male Army soldiers and marines who completed a Post-Deployment Health Assessment (PDHA) between May 1, 2003, and April 30, 2004, on return from deployments to OEF, OIF, and other locations (e.g., Bosnia, Kosovo)	Females 32,500 Males 271,404	Observational; To determine the relationship between deployment to Iraq and Afghanistan and mental health care utilization during the first year after return and to evaluate lessons learned from the postemployment mental health screening effort, particularly the correlation between screening results and actual use of mental health services.	Screening positive for PTSD, major depression, or other mental health problems; referral for a mental health reason; use of mental health care services after returning from deployment; attrition from military services	(1) The prevalence rates of mental health problems and combat experiences were consistently higher following deployment to OIF than to OEF or other locations. Among OIF veterans, 23.6% of women reported a mental health concern compared with 18.6% of men. (2) Referral to mental health was strongly correlated with screening positive for a mental health problem on the PDHA. Hospitalization was significantly associated with deployment location and reporting a mental health concern on the PDHA. (3) OIF veterans used inpatient and outpatient mental health services at higher rates after deployment than OEF veterans and service members who deployed to other locations.

Author	Sample Characteristics	Sample Size	Design/Objective	Main Measures	Main Findings
Hynes 2007[109]	National sample of veterans who were eligible to use VA and Medicare health care in calendar year 1999.	Females 37817 Males 1,436,600	Observational; To examine the impact of access to care characteristics on health care use patterns among those veterans dually eligible for Medicare and Veterans Affairs (VA) services.	Availability of health care resources, healthcare utilization; and cost; other factors included patient characteristics (age, gender, race, vital status), VA priority level, patient health status, distance to nearest VA facility, and demographic setting.	Multivariable analysis revealed that veterans who were black or had a higher VA priority were most likely to rely on the VA. Patient with higher risk scores were most likely to rely on a combination of VA and Medicare health care. Patients who lived farther from VA hospitals were less likely to rely on VA health care, particularly for inpatient care. Patients living in urban areas with more health care resources were less likely to rely on VA health care. Male veterans were less likely to rely exclusively on VA care than female veterans and less likely overall to rely on some VA care.
Kaplowitz 2006[134]	Female and male veterans at least 20 years old who had used outpatient services in the VA New England Health Care System at least once between January 1998 and December 1999 and at least once between January 2000 and June 2001	Females 2744 Males 61,746	Observational; To examine the relationship between mental illness, health care utilization and rates of cholesterol testing	receipt of cholesterol testing; mental illness diagnosis; frequency of VA outpatient visits	Among veterans using VA outpatient services infrequently, those with mental illness were less likely than non-mentally ill control subjects to receive a cholesterol test during the study period (first quartile adjusted OR [aOR]=0.45, 95% CI 0.37–0.54; second quartile aOR=0.50, 95% CI 0.45–0.57). Mentally ill subjects with more frequent utilization of VA services were as likely as (third quartile aOR=1.01, 95% CI 0.91–1.13) or more likely than (fourth quartile aOR=2.73, 95% CI=2.46–3.03) non-mentally ill subjects to receive cholesterol testing. Mental illness was associated with a lower likelihood of cholesterol testing in subjects who used fewer VA outpatient services. The observed disparity attenuated at higher levels of service utilization.

Author	Sample Characteristics	Sample Size	Design/Objective	Main Measures	Main Findings
Kaur 2007[115]	Female and male veterans at the Durham Veterans Affairs Medical Center between the ages of 21 and 60 that had two visits for the same pain location at least 6 weeks apart.	Females 406 Males 812	Observational; To identify differences in outpatient utilization between men and women veterans with chronic pain.	Visit data, number of pain sites, number of chronic pain conditions, comorbidity scores, and mental health diagnosis (depression, PTSD, substance abuse).	After adjusting for multiple pain sites, psychiatric diagnoses, age, and comorbidities, women veterans had a 27% higher rate of outpatient visits than men. Specifically, women had higher rates of visits to primary care, physical therapy, and other clinics, and had a higher rate of visits to address pain than did men. Women veterans with chronic pain may need more resources to adequately manage chronic pain conditions as well as associated comorbidities and psychiatric disease.
Kelly 2008[125]	National, cross-sectional sample of female veterans from the National Registry of Women Veterans stratified by age group, period of service, and race (black and non-black)	Females 1496	Observational; To investigate the effects of military sexual assault and combat exposure on women veterans' use of Veterans Health Administration (VHA) services and perceptions of VHA care.	Military sexual assault history, combat exposure, use of VHA services, satisfaction with VHA services	Women veterans with histories of military sexual assault reported more use of VHA services, but less satisfaction, poorer perceptions of VHA facilities and staff, and more problems with VHA services compared to women veterans without histories of sexual assault. Combat exposure was related to more problems with VHA staff, although few other differences were observed for women with and without histories of combat exposure.
Kimerling 2008[123]	Female and male veteran patients with valid positive or negative responses to military sexual trauma screening and at least one outpatient encounter 180 days before or after the screening date as identified by the VA Outpatient Events File	Females 33,259 Males 540,381	Observational; To evaluate the national efforts to screen for and treat military sexual trauma by prospectively examining rates of mental health utilization in 3-month period after screening.	Outpatient mental health services included specialized mental health or substance abuse treatment clinics; prescreen mental health care was 1 or more mental health visits in 6-months before the screening; postscreen mental health treatment was defined as 1 or more mental health visits in 3-months after screening.	Rates of positive screens were 19.5% for women and 1.2% for men. For both women and men, a positive military sexual trauma screen was associated with over twice the likelihood of postscreen mental health care, compared with negative screens. The number needed to screen to provide an impact number associated with the screening was one for every 5.5 positive screens in women and one for every 7.2 positive screens in men.

Author	Sample Characteristics	Sample Size	Design/Objective	Main Measures	Main Findings
Lairson 2005[119]	National random sample of female veterans 50 years or older taken from the National Registry of Women Veterans	Females 3415	Observational; To identify and measure the effect of economic, demographic, and behavioral factors that influence the use of mammography screening among US women veterans aged 50 and older	Mammography screening in the past year (15 month period used)	The findings included: about 75% of the women veteran respondents received a screening mammogram within the interval; and the demand models achieved a correct prediction for 75-77% of the sample. In the first model, increasing age, poor health, and smoking were inversely related to mammography use. In the second model, age, health status and income had smaller effects, and prior waiting time was inversely related to mammography screening in the past year.
Lang 2006[133]	Female veterans who received medical care from San Diego VA Healthcare System	Females 221	Observational; To examine whether current post-traumatic stress disorder (PTSD) mediates the relationship between exposure to childhood maltreatment (CM) and indicators of health and healthcare utilization in female veterans	Relationship between PTSD, exposure to childhood maltreatment (CM) and indicators of health and healthcare utilization	Increased emotional abuse ($\beta = -.32, p = .02$) was associated with poorer functioning on the SF-36 role-physical scale; increased emotional neglect ($\beta = .27, p = .02$) was associated with better functioning on the same scale. Higher levels of emotional abuse ($\beta = -.32, p = .01$) were associated with increased SF-36 bodily pain and greater odds of using pain medication in the past 6 months (OR = 1.14, $p = .01$). Greater physical abuse scores was associated with poorer SF-36 general health ($\beta = -.24, p = .04$), and CM was not associated with increased healthcare utilization. PTSD was shown to mediate the relationship between emotional and physical abuse and health outcomes.

Author	Sample Characteristics	Sample Size	Design/Objective	Main Measures	Main Findings
LaVela 2004[122]	Cross-sectional sample of veterans with SCI&D diagnoses identified from the Spinal Cord Dysfunction Registry (SCD-R) for 2001	Females 180 Males 8803	Observational; To describe inpatient (IP) and outpatient (OP) health care utilization of veterans with spinal cord injuries and disorders (SCI&D); to determine whether the health care utilization patterns of patients who reside at greater distances from their actual sources of care differ from those at shorter distances; to examine overall health care usage at the facility level to identify the types of VA facilities being used by SCI&D patients;	Inpatient and outpatient utilization	-Veterans with SCI&D utilized outpatient services less frequently when VA facilities were farther away from their residences (p<0.000). -Female, older, and non-white veterans (p<0.000 each), and veterans with a history of respiratory, kidney/urinary tract, circulatory, or digestive system diseases (p<0.005 for each) were more likely to use outpatient care during the study period. -History of prior illnesses, including respiratory, kidney/urinary tract, circulatory, digestive system, or skin/subcutaneous tissue or / breast-related illnesses (p<0.000 for each) were associated with greater likelihood of inpatient use.
LaVela 2006[113]	Female veteran data from a national cross-sectional survey mailed to Paralyzed Veterans of America (PVA) members for the SCI&D group and data from the CDC 2003 Behavioral Risk Factor Surveillance System (BRFSS) survey for the non-SCI&D comparison group	Females 593	Observational; To compare disease prevalence and preventive service use among female veterans in general and those with spinal cord injuries and disorders (SCI&D)	Disease/condition prevalence (asthma, diabetes, myocardial infarction, stroke, coronary heart disease, high blood pressure, high cholesterol, tooth decay/gum disease, injuries), health status (general health, physical and mental health), and use of preventive services (cholesterol check, dental care, influenza and pneumonia vaccinations, colon screening, breast and cervical cancer screening) among women veterans with and without SCI&D	Female veterans with SCI&D were similar in age and race but were better educated and less likely to be employed than female veterans in general. Coronary heart disease (CHD) prevalence was higher in those with SCI&D (17% vs. 8%, p < 0.0001). Health status was lower in SCI&D (27%) than in general female veterans (41%), p = 0.002. Fewer women with SCI&D, than female veterans in general reported having received recommended dental care (56% vs. 69%, p=0.004), colon screening in prior 5 years (59% vs. 72%, p = 0.023) or prior 10 years (67% vs. 92%, p < 0.0001), mammogram (84% vs. 91%, p = 0.019), and Pap smear (88% vs. 98%, p < 0.0001). There were no differences in receipt of respiratory vaccinations or cholesterol screening.

Author	Sample Characteristics	Sample Size	Design/Objective	Main Measures	Main Findings
Maguen 2007[139]	Female and male Vietnam veterans who served in the Vietnam theater of operations sometime between August 1964 and March 1975, who also participated in the National Vietnam Veterans Readjustment Study.	Females 432 Males 1200	Observational; To examine both direct and mediated relationships using predisposing factors, enabling factors, and need factors to predict medical and mental health care use for male and female veterans.	Predisposing variables (age, race, marital status, and combat exposure; enabling variables (family income, access to insurance); need variables (total number of psychiatric diagnoses, average number of physical health conditions, PTSD severity); service utilization variables (mental health care service utilization, physical health inpatient care utilization, physical health outpatient care utilization).	Need factors were the most consistent and strongest mediators of predisposing variables for both physical and mental health care service utilization, although there were differences between male and female veterans. For men, combat exposure indirectly predicted mental health care utilization through the need variables (with the effects of posttraumatic stress disorder being greatest). For women, physical health problems mediated the relationship between combat exposure and physical health outpatient care utilization.
McNulty 2005[25]	Female and male active duty Navy service members deployed on three aircraft carriers during OEF/OIF in 2002–2003	Females 259 Males 923	Observational; To describe the health care needs and perceived stressors of active duty members deployed to Iraq during the pre-deployment, mid-deployment, and postdeployment phases.	Member well-being, adaptation, coping, anxiety, stress, and health care needs	Logistic regression analyses indicated that many variables predicted extreme anxiety during deployment, including middeployment phase, age of under 25 years, being childless, nonattendance at church, being enlisted, zero- or one-deployment history; no high school education, and being currently in counseling. Active duty members in all phases of deployment had equally disturbing levels of anxiety. All phases reported suicidal ideation at alarming rates (2.4% in predeployment, 4.9% in middeployment, and 3% in postdeployment).

Author	Sample Characteristics	Sample Size	Design/Objective	Main Measures	Main Findings
Miller 2006[132]	National sample of female and male VA users during FY 2000 with no evidence of nursing home treatment during FY 1999 or FY 2000, followed through FY 2003 using administrative claims data.	Females 17096 Males 206,760	Observational; To determine whether patients with mental health diagnoses in the Department of Veterans Affairs (VA) are more likely to be admitted to nursing homes and to identify sociodemographic, utilization, and clinical characteristics associated with nursing home admission	Relationship between number of diagnosed mental illnesses and the risk of being admitted to a nursing home	Among mentally ill patients, risk of admission was highest for those with any inpatient medical/surgical days (odds ratio [OR] 2.28, 95% confidence interval [CI] 2.13-2.43), followed by 3+ outpatient medical visits (OR 1.48, 95% CI 1.42-1.55), inpatient mental health days (OR 1.31, 95% CI 1.22-1.40), and outpatient mental health visits (OR 1.09, 95% CI 1.02-1.18). Patients diagnosed with dementia were 58% more likely to be admitted. Patients admitted to nursing homes were more likely to be older ($P < 0.0001$), men ($P < 0.0001$), white ($P < 0.0001$), single ($P < 0.0001$), had higher incomes ($P < 0.0001$), and suffered from greater service-related disability ($P < 0.0001$).
Mojtabi 2003[138]	Female and male sample from National Collaborative Study of Early Psychosis and Suicide and comprised of U.S. Armed Forces personnel who had their first admission for major depression, bipolar disorder, or schizophrenia to a DoD hospital and were subsequently discharged from military services.	Females 754 Males 2106	Observational; To examine the use of Department of Veterans Affairs (VA) aftercare services among patients with serious mental disorders who were discharged from the military after a first admission to the Department of Defense (DoD) hospital.	Predictors of contact with VA versus no contact, and time to contact for those that do contact services.	Fifty-two percent of 2,861 identified individuals had received outpatient care from VA mental health clinics by the end of September 1998. Women, older persons, and persons with schizophrenia or bipolar disorder were more likely to contact VA outpatient mental health services than men, younger persons, and those with major depression. Also, being female, older than 25 years at military separation and having a diagnosis of bipolar disorder or schizophrenia were predictors of contacting services: women were more likely than men to use services.

Systematic Review of Women Veterans Health Research 2004-2008

Author	Sample Characteristics	Sample Size	Design/Objective	Main Measures	Main Findings
Mooney 2007[108]	Female veterans enrolled in the VA system who had an inpatient admission between 1998 and 2000 in either the VA or the private sector	Females 1409	Observational; To explore women veterans' use of Veterans Administration (VA) and private sector inpatient services	VA and private sector hospital admissions, length of stay (LOS), and method of payment for private sector care	Women admitted to the VA were less likely to be 65 or older (34% vs. 51%; p <.001); of those older women, those admitted to the VA were less likely to be enrolled in Medicare (87% vs. 96%, p <.001). Patients were less likely to be admitted to the VA for issues related to the female reproductive system (adjusted OR, 0.58; 95% CI, 0.39-0.87), the nervous system (adjusted OR, 0.64; 95% CI, 0.41- 0.99), the musculoskeletal system (adjusted OR, 0.72; 95% CI, 0.52-1.02), or the digestive system (adjusted OR, 0.77; 95% CI, 0.52-1.14). In contrast, patients were more likely to be admitted to the VA for alcohol or drug use (adjusted OR, 2.79; 95% CI, 1.57-4.95), mental diseases (adjusted OR, 2.1; 95% CI, 1.46-2.89), or care related to the skin/sub-cutaneous tissue and breasts (adjusted OR, 1.7; 95% CI, 0.99-2.92). Mean observed LOS were longer in the VA system for every diagnosis examined (but only reached statistical significance for mental, musculoskeletal, and nervous system disorders) despite comparable or even lower levels of acuity.
Nelson 2007[107]	National sample of veterans from the 2000 Behavioral Risk Factor Surveillance System	Females 1309 Males 22,488	Observational; To examine veteran reliance on health services provided by the VA and to describe the characteristics of veterans who receive VA care and report rates of uninsurance among veterans and characteristics of uninsured veterans.	use of VA health care, socio-demographic characteristics, access to care, health status, and health insurance coverage	Among veteran respondents, 6.2% reported re-ceiving all of their health care at the VA, 6.9% reported receiving some of their health care at the VA, and 86.9% did not use VA health care. Poor, less-educated, and minority veterans were more likely to receive all of their health care at the VA. Veterans younger than age 65 who used the VA for all of their health care also reported coverage with either private insurance (42.6%) or Medicare (36.3%). Of the veterans younger than age 65, 8.6% (population esti-mate 1.3 million individuals) were uninsured. Uninsured veterans were less likely to be able to afford a doctor or see a doctor within the year preceding the study.

Author	Sample Characteristics	Sample Size	Design/Objective	Main Measures	Main Findings
Polusny 2008[124]	Female veterans completing an anonymous cross-sectional survey and enrolled in an outpatient VA clinic.	Females 456	Observational; To examine the difficulties Identifying one's emotions (alexithymia) in understanding the link between PTSD symptoms and negative health outcome in sexually victimized female veterans	Physical health complaints, VA urgent healthcare utilization, sexual trauma exposure (Traumatic Life Events Questionnaire; TLEQ), PTSD symptom severity, and alexithymia (Toronto Alexithymia Scale; TAS-II)	A total of 57.5% reported a lifetime history of sexual trauma; 45.8% reported sexual trauma before age 18; and 32.2% reported sexual trauma after age 18. Hierarchial regression analyses showed that alexithymia independently explained unique variance in participants physical health and their visits to urgent care. These data suggest that emotion recognition problems may contribute to poorer heath outcome in sexually traumatized women veterans beyond what is explained by sexual trauma exposure, health risk behaviors and PTSD. Psychological interventions that enhance emotion identification skills for women who have experienced sexual trauma could improve health perceptions and reduce need for acute health care.
Ross 2008[104]	Nationally-representative sample of female and male community-dwelling adults, age 18 years or older, in 2004 Behavior Risk Factor Surveillance System	Females 422 Males 7569	Observational; To examine whether use of recommended ambulatory care services differs between exclusive and dual VA users	Self-reported use of 18 recommended services for cancer prevention, cardiovascular risk reduction, diabetes management, and infectious disease prevention	-Dual users were significantly more likely to be older and white, have higher incomes, have graduated from college, and be insured when compared with exclusive VA users. -After adjustment for patient characteristics, use of recommended services was largely similar among exclusive and dual VA users. -Exclusive VA users reported 14% greater use of breast cancer screening and 10% greater use of cholesterol monitoring among patients with hypercholesterolemia, and 6% lower use of prostate cancer screening and 7% lower use of influenza vaccination. -After adjustment for patient characteristics, exclusive and dual VA users reported similar rates of recommended ambulatory service use.

Author	Sample Characteristics	Sample Size	Design/Objective	Main Measures	Main Findings
Rowan 2006[140]	Female and male active duty Air Force Service Members seen in 8 outpatient mental health clinics during a 1-year period	Females 393 Males 812	Observational; To examine whether self-referred service members (SMs) are more likely to complete treatment than service members (SMs) referred by supervisors or those undergoing commander-directed evaluations.	Referral source (self, superiors encourages, commander directed), rank, special duty status, diagnostic category, treatment status, recommendations	Results showed significant differences across all variables, with self-referred members being more likely to be older, single, higher ranking, and without special duty status, as well as to have a less significant axis I diagnosis. Self-referred members were less likely to have confidentiality broken and to have career-affecting recommendations made. The implications of these findings, in terms of targeting interventions to increase self-initiated help-seeking behavior, and recommendations for future research are discussed.
Sadler 2005[127]	Stratified random sample of female veterans drawn from a historical national cohort who served in Vietnam, post-Vietnam, or Persian Gulf War eras from VA comprehensive women's health care registries.	Females 540	Observational; To determine whether there were differences in women veteran's health status and use of health care services by type of rape (gang, repeated, single, none) that occurred during military service	use of health care services and health status	Women who experience severe violence during their military service (repeated or gang rape) had significantly impaired physical and emotional health compared with women with a single or no rape (p≤.05). More than a decade after rape during military service, repeatedly raped women were more likely to use inpatient and outpatient mental health services than were women who experienced no rape or a single rape (p≤.05). Gang-rape survivors reported the most severe impairment in physical functioning and general health and demonstrated a trend to seek outpatient medical services.
Shen 2008[103]	National random mail survey of female and male veteran VA enrollees	Females 3440; Males 45,008	Observational; To examine private insurance coverage and its impact on use of Veterans Health Administration (VA) care among VA enrollees without Medicare coverage	Use of VA care by insurance status, insurance model (probability of having private insurance), comparisons of insurance effect in different models	- VA enrollees with private insurance coverage were less likely to use VA care. - Security selection dominated preference selection and naive models that did not control for selection effects consistently underestimated the insurance effect.

Author	Sample Characteristics	Sample Size	Design/Objective	Main Measures	Main Findings
Shen 2005[110]	Medicare-VA dual enrollees with full-year Part B coverage who completed the 1999 National Health Survey of Veterans Enrollees were included	Females 2167 Males 93,559	Observational; To examine the association between Veterans Administration (VA)-Medicare dual beneficiaries' HMO enrollment and factors including sociodemographics, access/attachment to VA, self-reported health status, and characteristics of Medicare HMO markets.	VA-Medicare dual beneficiaries' HMO enrollment	Dual beneficiaries' aged 65-69; those without college education; and those with VA Priority 5 (low income), 2 and 3 (with less than 50 percent service-connected disability) were more likely to enroll into Medicare HMOs. There was some evidence of favorable selection measured by self-reported health status. Availability of Medicare HMOs and less access to VA care were the major predictors of VA-Medicare dual beneficiaries' Medicare HMO enrollment.
Sherman 2005[118]	Random sample of female and male veteran smokers in primary care at 18 VA sites in the southwestern and western United States	Females 129 Males 1812	Observational; To examine if 1) there are gender differences among smokers using the Veterans Health Administration (VA) by sociodemographics, health and functional status, and health habits and 2) if there are gender differences in smoking cessation services received within the VA after adjusting for confounding factors.	Receipt of smoking cessation care, including: (a) Doctor or nurse talked about quitting smoking within last year; (b) Doctor referred me to a smoking cessation program within in last year; (c) Attended smoking cessation program within last year; (d) Doctor prescribed patches or nicotine gum within last year	Female smokers were younger, more educated, and less likely to be married than male smokers. Women were equally likely to report being advised to quit smoking or referred to a smoking cessation program but were much less likely to report receiving a prescription for nicotine patches (OR 0.5, 95% CI 0.3-0.9). One year later, female smokers were less likely to have successfully quit smoking.
Sherman 2005[136]	Sample veterans (and their female partners) who served in the Vietnam War, had a diagnosis of PTSD and service-connected disability for PTSD, participated in the PTSD program, and current cohabitation with a female partner recruited from two VA medical centers.	Females 72	Observational; To perform an initial needs assessment of partners of Vietnam veterans with combat-related post-traumatic stress disorder (PTSD) and to assess the partners' current rates of treatment use.	Partner treatment experiences and ratings of treatment needs; partners' assessment of her need for individual treatment and the partner's appraisal of family treatment being extremely important (yes/no).	Although large majorities of partners rated individual (64%) and family therapy (78%) to help cope with PTSD in the family as extremely or very important, only 28% had received any mental health care in the previous six months. Significant predictors of desire for individual treatment included partner's anxiety and patient-partner contact, and partner's age and severity of the patient's PTSD symptoms were significant predictors of family treatment. The most commonly requested service was a women-only group.

Author	Sample Characteristics	Sample Size	Design/Objective	Main Measures	Main Findings
Singh 2007[114]	Female and male veterans who received medical care from an Upper Midwest Veterans Integrated Service Network (former VISN 13) facility between 10/1/96 and 3/31/98 and completed a mailed survey	Females 1500 Males 35,000	Observational: To compare women and men veterans' health-related quality of life (HRQOL) and VA health care utilization and to see if previously described associations between HRQOL, subsequent VA health care utilization, and mortality in male veterans would generalize to women veterans	HRQOL, VA health care utilization and mortality in the year after survey, gender-specific impact of HRQOL on VA health care utilization and on mortality in the year after the survey	Women's effective survey response rate was 52%, men's 58%. In the following year, 9% of women and 12% of men had at least one hospitalization. One percent of women and 3% of men died in the post-survey year. After adjustment, women's HRQOL was higher than men's; for every 10-point decrement in overall physical or mental functioning, women and men had similarly increased risk/odds of subsequently dying, being hospitalized at a VA facility, or making a VA outpatient stop. Among younger women and women who received VA care outside of the Twin City metro area, poorer overall mental or physical health functioning was associated with few primary care stops; among their male counterparts, it was associated with more primary care stops.
Stein 2004[128]	Female patient sample in VA San Diego Healthcare System (VASDHS) primary care outpatient clinic.	Females 219	Observational; To determine whether there is an association between sexual assault history and measures of somatic symptoms and illness attitudes in a sample of female Veterans Affairs primary care patients, a group in whom high rates of sexual trauma have been reported.	Traumatic exposure, including sexual assault, physical complaints, healthcare utilization, reported sick days, somatization symptoms, health anxiety.	Sexual assault was associated with a significant increase in somatization scores, physical complaints across multiple symptom domains and health anxiety. Sexual assault was also a significant statistical predictor of having multiple sick days in the prior 6 months and of being a high utilizer of primary care visits in the prior 6 months. These data confirm a strong association between sexual trauma exposure and somatic symptoms, illness attitudes and healthcare utilization in women.
Vogt 2006[101]	Nationally representative sample of female veterans who used VA care (i.e., current and former users) and were a subset of National Registry of Women Veterans	Females: 942	Observational; To document perceived and/ or actual barriers to care in a nationally representative sample of female veterans and examine associations with VA use.	Ratings of VA care and care in other facilities; ratings of barriers to VA care (i.e., availability of services, physician sensitivity and skill, logistics of care, and facility/ physical environment characteristics).	The greatest barrier to the use of VA care was problems related to ease of use. In the model with background characteristics plus all 4 barrier domains, only availability of services (OR 0.49, 95%CI 0.29-0.80) and facility/physical environment characteristics remained (OR 1.93, 95%CI 1.16-3.19) retained significant associations with VA use.

Author	Sample Characteristics	Sample Size	Design/Objective	Main Measures	Main Findings
Wakefield 2007[106]	Female and male veteran VA users and nonusers from one Midwestern VAMC	Females 7 Males 35	Observational; To examine veterans' perceptions of problems and benefits of outsourcing inpatient care from Veterans Affairs (VA) hospitals to private sector hospitals.	reasons veterans choose whether or not to use VA services	The focus groups identified six domains related to why veterans use or do not use VA services; cost, access, quality of care, contract (i.e., covenant between veterans and the U.S. government), veteran milieu, special needs. With the exception of veteran milieu, these same domains were identified with regard to the potential positive and negative impacts of outsourcing inpatient care to non-VA hospitals; two additional outsourcing domains were also identified, choice and discrimination. Cost was the first reason veterans gave for using the VA; access and quality were In general, veterans perceived more advantages than disadvantages to outsourcing VA care but still expressed significant concerns related to outsourcing.
Washington 2007[51]	VA-eligible women veterans in Los Angeles, California formed 6 focus groups: 4 with women who used VA health care (VA users) and 2 with women who have never used or have not used VA in the past 5 years (nonusers)	Females 51	Observational; To determine women veterans' perspectives and decision-making about VA health care use	Patient reported themes on information needs, access, gender appropriateness of services and gender-related aspects of care, quality of care	Barriers to VA use for both VA users and nonusers included lack of information about eligibility and available services. Nonusers often assumed the VA did not provide women's health care. All groups emphasized they required a health care system focused on quality and sensitivity to women's health issues. However, users and nonusers differed in perceptions of VA quality. VA environment and quality concerns led many women to limit their VA use to women's clinics.

Author	Sample Characteristics	Sample Size	Design/Objective	Main Measures	Main Findings
Washington 2006[102]	Female veterans who participated in a cross-sectional telephone survey of 2,174 VA users and VA-eligible non-users	Females 2174	Observational; To determine why women veterans use or do not use VA health care	Reasons for choice of VA versus non-VA health care setting, knowledge and perceptions of VA, independent predictors of type of ambulatory care use, demographics and health status	Reasons cited for VA use included affordability (67.9%); women's health clinic (WHC) availability (58.8%); quality of care (54.8%); and convenience (47.9%). Reasons for choosing health care in non-VA settings included having insurance (71.0%); greater convenience of non-VA care (66.9%); lack of knowledge of VA eligibility and services (48.5%); and perceived better non-VA quality (34.5%). After adjustment for sociodemographics, health characteristics, and VA priority group, knowledge deficits about VA eligibility and services and perceived worse VA care quality predicted outside health care use.
Washington 2006[46]	National sample of VA sites serving 400 or more women veterans in fiscal year 2000	Nonpatient 118	To assess the availability of women's health care specialists for emergency gynecological problems (GYN) and for emergency mental health conditions specific to women (WMH).	Availability of women's health care specialists for emergency gynecologic problems (GYN) and emergency mental health (MH) conditions specific to women during clinic hours and after hours.	-The majority of sites had GYN and MH specialists available for emergencies during clinic hours (64.4% and 82.7% of sites, respectively). -Availability of specialists after hours for GYN emergencies was 39.8%, for MH emergencies was 51.7%. -Two significant predictors: separate women's health clinic was associated with availability of emergency GYN services (beta: 0.279, p=0.023), and lower local managed care penetration was associated with availability of emergency MH conditions specific to women (beta: -0.282, p=0.024).
Zeber 2007[105]	Secondary data on Female and male veterans contained in the National Psychoses Registry from June 1, 2000, through September 30, 2003, for all veterans diagnosed with schizophrenia and receiving healthcare through the Department of Veterans Affairs.	Females 4275 Males 76,393	Observational; To assess the effect of the 200 Veterans Millennium Health Care Act, which raised pharmacy copayments from $2 to $7 for lower-priority patients, on medication refill decisions and health services utilization among vulnerable veterans with schizophrenia	total prescription fills, medical and psychotropic fills separately, outpatient visits, psychiatric admission, inpatient days among those admitted, and pharmacy costs	Total prescriptions and overall pharmacy costs leveled among veterans with copayments after the medication cost increase. However, psychiatric drug refills dropped substantially, nearly 25%. Although outpatient visits were unaffected, psychiatric admissions and total inpatient days increased slightly, particularly 10-20 months after the policy change.

Author	Sample Characteristics	Sample Size	Design/Objective	Main Measures	Main Findings
Zinzow 2008[126]	Random sample of female and male primary care users at one of four Veterans Affairs Medical Centers (Charleston or Columbia, SC; Tuscaloosa or Birmingham, AL)	Female 173 Male 816	Observational; To examine the nature and prevalence of sexual assault (SA), as well as its relationship to psychiatric sequelae and service use, among the veteran population	Sexual assault characteristics, trauma history, psychiatric diagnoses and global health functioning, service use	-Lifetime prevalence of SA was 38% among women and 6% among men. Of veterans reporting a history of SA, most experienced child sexual abuse and sexual re-victimization. -SA victims had a more extensive trauma history and demonstrated greater psychological impairment in comparison to veterans reporting other types of trauma. -Only 25% of male SA survivors and 38% of female SA survivors used mental health services in the past year.

APPENDIX 9. PSYCHIATRIC/MENTAL HEALTH ISSUES EVIDENCE TABLE

Author	Sample Characteristics	Sample Size	Design/Objective	Main Measures	Main Findings
2007[28]	Female and male service members who deployed to OIF and completed post deployment health assessments (PDHA) and possibly post deployment health reassessments (PDHRA)	23,194 Females 198,989 Males	Observational; To document the frequencies of self-reported symptoms of and provider referrals during PDHAs among service members who subsequently showed evidence of PTSD	Responses to PTSD-related questions of PDHA's and medical referral experiences of Operation Iraqi Freedom (OIF) deployers who were diagnosed with PTSD within six months after return from deployment; and/or screened positive for PTSD on Post Deployment Health Reassessment (PDHRA) questionnaires.	-Among PDHA respondents, 24.9% were referred for health concerns of any type, 10.5% screened positive for PTSD, and 4.1% were referred for mental health concerns. Among PDHA respondents who were clinically diagnosed with PTSD within six months after deployment (n=2676), 54.7% had been referred for a health concern, 48.1% had screened positive for PTSD, and 27.0% had been referred for a mental health concern during their PDHAs. -Females were more likely than males to receive referrals for health concerns in general and for mental health concerns specifically. -However, females were not more likely to screen positive for PTSD during PDHAs. Female and male clinically diagnosed cases and possible cases (per PDHRA responses) of PTSD had a similar prevalence of screening positive for PTSD on their PDHA questionnaire.
Asmundson 2004[49]	Female veterans obtaining general medical consults at one VA	Females 221	Observational; To evaluate the co-occurrence of pain and PTSD symptoms among women veterans.	PTSD symptoms using the PTSD Checklist Civilian version (PCL-C)	-Pain-related variables were significant predictors of PTSD symptom cluster scores, including bodily pain, bothered by severe headache or migraine, and pain interference, as well as childhood trauma scores. -The PTSD group had significantly higher values compared to the no PTSD group, and with the exception of bodily pain, the subsyndromal PTSD group had significantly higher values than the no PTSD group. -Childhood trauma, pain interference, experience of sexual assault in the military and being bothered by severe headache or migraine were significant predictors of the re-experiencing symptoms. -Childhood trauma, pain interference and experience of sexual assault in the military were significant predictors of avoidance/numbing symptoms and hyperarousal symptoms.

Author	Sample Characteristics	Sample Size	Design/Objective	Main Measures	Main Findings
Becker 2006[152]	Outpatient and inpatient female veterans who received treatment at the Durham VAMC.	Females 236	Observational; To examine the effect of childhood risk/trauma indicators and the secondary effect of combat exposure in contributing to PTSD, depression, substance abuse and physical health status	Family loss and instability measured by the childhood events scale, childhood physical abuse, childhood sexual abuse, and combat exposure effect on PTSD symptom severity and physical health outcomes.	Socio-demographic variables did not explain any of the dependent variables. Childhood physical and sexual abuse were significantly associated with PTSD symptom severity, while family loss/instability and childhood physical abuse were positively associated with negative physical health status. However, no effects were found linking childhood adversity variables with depression or substance abuse. Additionally, combat exposure did not show a mediating or moderating role regarding its relationship to childhood adversity or physical health status.
Benda 2005[168]	Convenience sample of all homeless female veterans that entered an inpatient VA domiciliary program for substance abuse in a 3-year period. Systematic random sample of homeless men that entered program during same period.	Females 310 Males 315	Observational; (1) to study gender differences in predictors of readmission to inpatient drug treatment among homeless veterans because VA medical centers currently do not have services that are designed specifically for women; (2) are abuses at different stages of life span, combat exposure, and recent traumatic evens commensurate predictors, do employment, housing, family or friend relationships and spirituality mediate (3) or moderate (4) relationships between trauma and relapse.	Re-admission to inpatient drug treatment in a two-year follow-up.	-Sexual and physical abuse in childhood or during active duty in the military and during the past 2 years were most potent predictors of readmission for women than men. Women's readmission was heightened by increases in depression, suicidal thoughts, and traumatic events. Women's readmission was lessened by greater family, friend, church or other support. -Men's readmission increased with greater substance abuse, aggression, and cognitive impairment. Men's readmission decreases with employment stability and job satisfaction.
Berz 2008[156]	Female veterans of the Vietnam war who had biological children who were a subgroup of the National Vietnam Veterans Readjustment Survey and had participated in the family interview component.	Females 60	Observational; To examine the relationships between the posttraumatic stress disorder (PTSD) symptom clusters and parenting satisfaction in female Vietnam veterans.	Parenting satisfaction	In the multiple regression models, hyperarousal was the only symptom cluster which showed a significant and negative relationship with parenting satisfaction (p=.02). No other cluster had an effect.

112

Author	Sample Characteristics	Sample Size	Design/Objective	Main Measures	Main Findings
Brailey 2007[153]	Female and male active duty Army soldiers	Females 158 Males 1421	Observational; To describe risk and resilience factors potentially impacting troops prior to warzone deployment. Specifically, demographic, stressor exposure variables, and situational factors were measured in a large cohort of Army soldiers who had not yet been deployed to either OIF or OEF. As a situational factor, we focused on unit cohesion, a contextual military variable.	PTSD Checklist, Deployment Risk and Resilience Inventory, military unit cohesion	Regression analysis revealed that life experiences and unit cohesion strongly and independently predicted PTSD symptoms, and that unit cohesion attenuated the impact of life experiences on PTSD. Some military personnel reported significant pre-deployment, stress-related symptoms. These symptoms may serve as vulnerabilities that could potentially be activated by subsequent war-zone deployment. Higher pre-deployment unit cohesion levels appear to ameliorate such symptoms, potentially lessening future vulnerability.
Busch 2004[77]	Female and male veteran VA users and non-VA population of employees and retirees with depression diagnosis and initiation of antidepressants	*3028 VA Females 24,685 VA Males 3295 Non-VA Females 1557 Non-VA Males	Observational; To compare quality of pharmacotherapy for patients with major depression in the VA and the private sector	Quality of depression care pharmacotherapy (HEDIS measure of antidepressant medication management, e.g., proportion of patients with 3 or more follow-up office visits in 12 weeks after depression diagnosis)	-More than 80% of patients who began antidepressant treatment achieved guideline-level acute-phase treatment. -Few differences in the quality of pharmacotherapy for depression were found between VA and the private sector, with VA slightly outperforming in prescription of antidepressants during acute (84.7% vs. 81.0%) and maintenance phases of treatment (53.9% vs. 50.9%). -Patient characteristics associated with pharmacotherapy quality included being female, and having a comorbid diagnosis of substance use, bipolar disorder, or anxiety or adjustment disorder.
Butterfield 2001[7]	Female and male veteran and nonveteran patients ages 18-70 years with criteria for PTSD recruited from Duke University Outpatient Psychiatry Center and VA Durham Comprehensive Women's Health Center	Females 14 Males 1	Experimental; To evaluate olanzapine efficacy and tolerance over 10 weeks compared to placebo in noncombat PTSD patients	Compliance with dose, treatment related events reported, Barnes Akathisia Scale (BAS), abnormal involuntary movement scale (AIMS) weight gain, psychometric measures, PTSD assessments with multiple measures	Patients in both groups showed improvements in PTSD symptoms, but no between group differences in treatment response were observed and a high placebo response was found.

Author	Sample Characteristics	Sample Size	Design/Objective	Main Measures	Main Findings
Campbell 2008[164]	Female veterans or reservists from a VA hospital women's clinic in a large Midwestern city.	Females 268	Observational; To examine the co-occurrence of childhood sexual abuse (CSA), adult sexual assault (ASA), intimate partner violence (IPV), and sexual harassment (SA) in a predominantly low-income, African American female veteran sample, and the detrimental impact of that collective violence on their mental and physical health.	Four forms of violence; CSA, ASA, IPV, SA; and Post-Traumatic Stress symptomatology (PTS)	African-American female veterans were found to have experienced more violence than their Caucasian military counterparts, but their experiences are not markedly different than other low-income African-American women.
Copeland 2008[198]	Female and male inpatients and outpatients sequentially recruited into the Continuous Improvement for Veterans in Care—Mood Disorders at one VA medical center.	Females 61 Males 373	Observational; To determine the association of insight and adherence in a large sample of VA patients with bipolar disorder, controlling for potentially confounding patient factors, to identify modifiable factors to improve care for these patients.	Scales comprised 8 questions in 2 domains to assess belief in the likelihood that medications or psychotherapy would be effective in achieving treatment goals, such as symptom relief and relapse prevention. Socio-demographic factors, medication adherence (2 measures), substance use, symptoms, and service-connected status were also assessed.	Among 435 patients with bipolar disorder, 27% had poor adherence based on missed dose and 46% had poor adherence based on the Morisky scale. In multivariable models, greater insight into medication was negatively associated with both measures of poor adherence. Odds of poor adherence increased for women, African Americans, mania, and hazardous drinking. The association of mutable factors—hazardous drinking, manic symptoms, and insight— could represent an opportunity to improve adherence.
David (2006)[5]	Female veterans with PTSD at 1 VA clinic	Females 10	Clinical Trial; Evaluation of 12-week open trial of behavioral intervention with structured group psycho education and self-defense training. (All participants received the intervention.)	Risk perception of assault, psychiatric symptoms (i.e., PTSD, depression, anxiety, and hostility scales), and specific self-efficacy parameters (i.e., general, interpersonal, activities, and self-defense scales) were measured at 5 time points	Significant and sustained improvement at 3 and 6 months after program for PTSD avoidance behavior and hyperarousal symptoms, decreased depression scores, and increased interpersonal self-efficacy, self defense self-efficacy, and willingness to participate in community activities

Author	Sample Characteristics	Sample Size	Design/Objective	Main Measures	Main Findings
David (2004)[184]	Female veterans with physical or sexual assault histories receiving outpatient mental health services at an urban VA clinic	Females 64	Observational; To ascertain beliefs about the potential value of personal safety/self defense training among women veterans with a history of physical or sexual assault.	Beliefs about value of personal safety/self-defense training	1. Most traumatized female veterans believe that personal safety/self-defense training would be an effective and powerful addition to more traditional treatments for PTSD. 2. Study participants indicated they believe such training would positively affect their sense of personal safety, promote increased competence in thwarting future assaults, improve their self-esteem, confidence and assertiveness, and reduce avoidant and agoraphobic behaviors.
Desai (2006)[197]	Female and male national sample of VA medical outpatients with no depression diagnosis or mental health visits in the past 6 months	Females 3646 Males 17843	Observational; To determine the rates and predictors of screening, screening positive, follow-up evaluation, and subsequent diagnosis of depression among medical outpatients.	(1) screened for depression in the outpatient setting, (2) among those screened, the proportion who screened positive according to standard, instrument specific cutoffs, (3) among those screened positive, whether the patient received follow-up evaluation within 6 weeks, and (4) among those followed up, the proportion who received a depressive disorder diagnosis according to the External Peer Review Program (EPRP) chart review.	Overall, 84.9% of eligible patients (n=18,245) were screened for depression in the past year. Of the 8.8% who screened positive, only 54% received follow-up evaluation, and of these, 23.6% (n=204) subsequently were diagnosed with a depressive disorder. Patients who were younger, unmarried, and had more medical comorbidities were less likely to be screened; however, if screened, they were more likely to screen positive. Male gender and greater medical comorbidity were associated with decreased odds of follow-up evaluation after a positive screen.
Desai (2005)[58]	Female and male VA patient respondents to the National VA Customer Feedback Survey, identified as having a visit to a VA general medicine, primary care, or women's clinic between March 1 - April, 23, 1999, who were not admitted to the hospital in the same time period	Females 5170 Males 45362	Observational; The objective of this study was to assess the role of psychiatric illness in satisfaction with outpatient primary care services in the VA.	core satisfaction with healthcare, including overall coordination of care among providers; open sharing of information with the patient; timeliness and accessibility of service; courtesy of staff; emotional support; coordination of care; specialist provider access; pharmacy access; and continuity of care	After controlling for patient characteristics (e.g., gender, age, disability, acute vs. routine visit) and subjective health, patients with schizophrenia, post-traumatic stress disorder, drug abuse, depression, and other psychiatric disorders reported significantly lower satisfaction with their outpatient primary care. Dissatisfaction was particularly reported for access to care and overall coordination of care.

Author	Sample Characteristics	Sample Size	Design/Objective	Main Measures	Main Findings
Dobie (2006)[129]	Female veterans receiving care between 10/01/1996 - 1/01/2000 at VA Puget Sound Health Care System	Females 2578	Observational; To determine associations between medical/surgical utilization and PTSD in female patients	Rates of medical/surgical hospitalizations, surgical inpatient procedures, and outpatient utilization for PTSD positive and PTSD negative women.	Female veterans who screen positive for PTSD receive more VA medical/surgical services. About 33% of the women screened positive for PTSD. PTSD+ women had higher rates of medical/surgical hospitalizations of 20% vs. 14% overall. In particular, PTSD+ women ages 35-49 had significantly more mean hospital days compared to PTSD- women (43 vs. 17 days, p<.0001). Similarly, more PTSD+ women ages 35-49 underwent surgical procedures (5.9% vs. 1.7%, p<.001). Mean annual outpatient visits were also significantly higher among PTSD+ women (p<.001 for each comparison).
Dobie 2004[160]	Female clinic patients who received care at the VA Puget Sound Healthcare System	Females 1209	To identify self-reported health problems and functional impairment associated with screening positive for PTSD in women in seen in VA	Screen positive PTSD symptomatology, lowest quartile SF36V mental and physical component scores	PTSD symptoms are common among women treated at VA facilities (22% screened positive). Screening positive was associated with younger age and separated/divorced status. PTSD is associated with multiple self-reported mental and physical health problems and poor health-related quality of life after adjustment for other patient characteristics.
Dove 2007[171]	Women admitted to the TRISARF (at the Pacific Regional Medical Command facility) for all chemically addicted Department of Defense-eligible beneficiaries between the ages of 18 and 64 years.	Females 86	Observational; To determine sociodemographic characteristics, coexisting conditions and referral sources of women in a substance use treatment center at a Pacific Regional Medical Command facility.	Admission to Tri-Service Addictions and Recovery Facility (TRISARF) for substance use treatment.	Except for educational level, the military population's sociodemographic characteristics did not differ from those of the general population. Seventy-eight percent reported a coexisting psychiatric condition, and the most frequently occurring conditions were depression and anxiety. Alcohol and nicotine were the two major substances of abuses with 76% and 85% respectively of the women's records showing use of these substances. The smallest number of referrals was from primary care managers.

Systematic Review of Women Veterans Health Research 2004-2008

Author	Sample Characteristics	Sample Size	Design/Objective	Main Measures	Main Findings
Erbes (2007)[15]	Female and male OEF/ OIF veteran enrollees (n=120) at one Midwestern VAMC who had returned within a six-month time frame, agreed to participate and completed a questionnaire	17 Females 103 Males	Observational; To evaluate levels of PTSD, depression, alcohol abuse, and the associations with quality of life, and mental health service utilization among returnees from OEF/OIF.	psychiatric distress levels (measured by PTSD symptoms, depression symptoms, and hazardous alcohol use), functional impairment, and service utilization	1. PTSD levels (12%) were consistent with previous research while problematic drinking levels were also elevated (33%) 2. PTSD and alcohol abuse were associated with lower quality of life in multiple domains, even when controlling for depression. 3. Of those screening positive for PTSD, 56% reported using mental health services. Only 18% of those screening positive for alcohol abuse reported using such services. 4. No reported findings were identified as related to gender.
Escalona (2004)[148]	Female veterans and non-veterans (i.e., veteran spouses) in one VA primary care clinic (Albuquerque, NM).	Females 294	Observational; To explore associations between trauma, PTSD and somatization among women in a VAMC primary care clinic	Patients were defined as somatizers if they med abridged somatization criteria based on responses to the presence of six unexplained somatic symptoms from 35 possible based on DSM-IV criteria for diagnosis	1. Traumatic events were reported by 81% of the women, with lifetime prevalence of PTSD at 27%, and somatization at 19%. 2. PTSD was the best predictor of somatization after controlling for demographic characteristics, veteran status and other mood and anxiety disorders. Of PTSD symptoms, psychological numbing was the strongest predictor of somatization.
Fontana 2006[135]	Female veterans with consecutive admissions to the Women's Stress Disorder Treatment Team (WSDTT) at 4 VA sites.	Females 224	Observational; To examine the role of women's comfort in coming for treatment of PTSD in a predominantly male environment	Female veterans comfort level when entering treatment and while participating in therapy, socio-demographic and clinical characteristics associated with comfort level, and strength of association of comfort level and participation and satisfaction with treatment.	(1) Women treated for military-related stress disorder were "somewhat comfortable" in coming to the VA for specialized PTSD treatment from the start. The most important factor contributing to their level of comfort was the availability of a specialized treatment program for women. (2) Women who had prior contact with the VA reported no change in comfort level over the 8-month period. Women who did not have prior contact with the VA reported an increase in comfort from intake to 4 months. (3) Among women who did not have prior contact with the VA, those of minority ethnicity had significantly lower comfort levels, and, among women who did have prior contact with the VA, those with higher levels of education had significantly lower comfort levels. (4) Comfort level did not have a significant effect on their satisfaction with treatment.

Author	Sample Characteristics	Sample Size	Design/Objective	Main Measures	Main Findings
Forman-Hoffman 2005[174]	Female and male active duty personnel in the first Gulf War who were part of the Iowa Gulf War Study Case Validation study	Females 73 Males 529	Observational; To examine the patterns of coexisting (comorbid) mental disorders and whether comorbidity influences quality of life ratings in a sample of U.S. veterans.	Mental disorders were defined using the SCID-IV, and the Health Utilities Index Mark 3 (HUI3) was used to measure health-related quality of life (HRQoL).	Over 35% of veterans with a current mental disorder had at least one other comorbid mental disorder. Those with mental disorder comorbidity had lower HUI scores than veterans with only one or less mental disorders (Mean 0.41 ± 0.30 vs. 0.72 ± 0.25, $p < 0.0001$.
Frayne 2006[179]	National random sample of veterans in Large Health Survey of Veteran Enrollees (1999), who were sent a mailed survey of health and functional status	Females 28048 Males 651811	Observational; To characterize the health status of women (vs men) veteran VA patients across age cohorts, and assess gender differences in the effect of social support on health status.	All eight domains of veterans short form (SF-36) health status survey, mental and physical component scores	Physical and mental component scores were similar by gender except among those age 65 or older, mean MCS was better for women than men (49.3 vs 45.9, $p<.001$). Patient gender had a clinically insignificant effect upon PCS and MCS after adjusting for age, race/ethnicity, and education. Women had lower levels of support than men: in patients aged<65, being married or living with someone benefited MCS more in men than in women.
Frayne 2004[162]	Female veterans in the 1999 Large Health Survey of Veteran Enrollees, with self reported history of PTSD, depression, or neither	Females 30865	To examine the number of medical symptoms and physical health status in women with PTSD across age strata and benchmark them against those of women with depression alone or with neither depression nor PTSD.	All 4 domains of the short form health status (SF-36V) scale used for physical health – physical functioning, role limitations due to physical problems, bodily pain, and energy/vitality	Across age strata, women with PTSD (n=4348) had more medical conditions and worse physical health status than women with depression alone (n=7580) or neither (n=18937). In age-adjusted analyses, the physical component summary score was on average, 3.4 points lower in women with depression alone and 6.3 points lower in women with PTSD than in women with neither (p<.001).

Author	Sample Characteristics	Sample Size	Design/Objective	Main Measures	Main Findings
Frueh 2007[131]	Random sample of female and male veterans less than 80 years old at 4 VAMC primary care clinics selected in fiscal year 1999	Females 50 Males 695	Observational; To expand our understanding of PTSD prevalence, its psychiatric characteristics, and service use among elderly veterans in VA primary care clinics	prevalence of PTSD and psychiatric diagnoses by age; physical and mental health functioning by age; use of VA mental health services and disability benefits; identification of explanatory characteristics	Those in the 45–64 year age group endorsed the highest scores and those in the oldest age group (65 and older) endorsed the lowest scores, even after adjusting for the effects of race and sex. Similarly, those in the oldest group (7.5%) had one-third of the prevalence of major depression as those in the two younger groups (21.7% and 22.9%), and they had a lower prevalence of other psychiatric conditions, such as panic disorder, agoraphobia, social anxiety, and substance abuse. They also were about half as likely to show evidence of suicidal risk. In all cases, these differences were maintained even after controlling for relevant demographic covariates, such as race and sex. Those in the 45–64 year old group were generally more likely to meet criteria for most psychiatric disorders, followed by the 18–44 group, and then the 65 and older group. All but one of these relationships remained significant after adjusting for the effects of race and sex. The one exception was in rates of substance abuse/dependence between the 45–64 and 65 and older groups.
Gahm 2007[161]	Female and male active duty personnel newly seen in a military outpatient mental health clinic between June 2003 and October 2004	Females 325 Males 1256	Observational; The purpose of this study is to determine the relative contributions of demographics and reported childhood and adulthood trauma on screened PTSD and depression symptoms for soldiers in a military outpatient mental health setting.	Symptoms of PTSD and Depression, adverse childhood events (ACE) items, deployment risk and resilience inventory	1) Univariate analyses indicated that more women met cutoff criteria for both PTSD and depression. Men more likely experienced a war or combat zone, witnessed an assault or kill, and to have been robbed. Women more likely experienced childhood sexual abuse than men. No gender differences in child physical abuse, witnessed parental violence, parental substance abuse, or experience of natural disaster occurred. 2) The regression model was significant for PTSD, with the experiences of combat (OR 2.09), witnessing someone being assaulted or killed (OR 1.88), and number of adverse childhood events (OR 1.25) emerging as significant risk factors. Witnessing someone being assaulted or killed (OR 1.56) and number of adverse childhood events (OR 1.34) significantly predicted screened depression status above demographic factors, but exposure to combat was not a significant predictor in this model.

Author	Sample Characteristics	Sample Size	Design/Objective	Main Measures	Main Findings
Gahm 2008[176]	Female and male active duty Army soldiers who entered an outpatient Behavioral Health (BH) clinic located in an Army medical treatment facility on a large military base	Females 555 Males 2313	Observational; To describe the mental health characteristics identified through screening of soldiers seeking care during time of war in a military outpatient mental health setting, using the Behavioral Health Screening Instrument (BHSI).	Findings on clinical scales (i.e. depression, anxiety, panic, PTSD, and alcohol use) and for demographic and psychological domains for soldiers seeking mental health services.	Average mean scores were significantly higher for women on the following clinical scales: panic, depression, anxiety, and hostility. Men had significantly higher levels of both unit support and relationship satisfaction (p<0.01). There were no gender differences detected on the mean PTSD scores. 89.4% of the total sample screened positive for at least one domain of behavioral health difficulty. Both men and women reported low levels of marital satisfaction, although the mean score was significantly higher for men. Overall marital satisfaction scores were lower for the active duty soldiers than that of a studied depressed civilian population.
Gielen 2006[192]	Female active duty personnel from all services	Females 474	Observational; To describe active duty military (ADM) women's beliefs and preferences concerning domestic violence (DV) policy in the military.	Beliefs about the consequences of routine screening and mandatory reporting; Policy preferences for routine screening and mandatory reporting	119 women had experienced DV during their military service. A majority (57%) supported routine screening. Although 87% said the military's policy on mandatory reporting should remain the same, only 48% thought abuse should be reported to the commanding officer; abused women were significantly less likely than non-abused women to agree with this aspect of the policy. ADM women's beliefs were similar to those of women in a previously studied civilian sample, except that 73% of ADM compared to 43% of civilian women thought routine screening would increase women's risk of further abuse.
Gold 2007[155]	Female veterans of the Vietnam war and their male relationship partners who were a subgroup of the National Vietnam Veterans Readjustment Survey and had participated in the family interview component	Females 89	Observational; This study examined relations between posttraumatic stress disorder (PTSD) symptom severity and several family adjustment variables among female Vietnam veterans.	Correlation between PTSD symptom severity and marital adjustment, family adaptability, family cohesion, parenting satisfaction, and abuse, well being, and child behavior	A negative and statistically significant correlation was found between female veteran's PTSD symptom severity and marital adjustment (r=-.38, p<.01), family adaptability (r=-.40, p<.01) and cohesion (r=-.34, p<.01) and parenting satisfaction (r=-.31, p<.01). However, for the male partner, PTSD symptom severity was only significantly correlated with male ratings of veteran's psychological abuse (r=.21, p=.02).

Author	Sample Characteristics	Sample Size	Design/Objective	Main Measures	Main Findings
Greenberg 2004[137]	Female veterans entering outpatient treatment for PTSD at one of 4 VA Women's Stress Disorders Treatment Programs (Boston, Brecksville, Loma Linda, New Orleans).	Females 149	Observational; To examine the strength of association of care and health outcomes for female veterans newly entering outpatient treatment for PTSD.	Changes in clinical status between program entry and four months follow-up on 11 measures (e.g., PTSD symptoms, general psychiatric/physical health, alcohol and drug abuse, violent behavior).	1. Few significant associations between continuity and outcomes were found. 2. Four months after program entry, only commitment to treatment (treatment process) was positively associated with one or more continuity of care measures. 3. Severity continuity of care measures were associated with poor health outcomes. 4. Eight months after program entry, patients with greater continuity of care during the first four months of treatment had greater declines in violent behavior and PTSD measurements and larger increases in global functioning. 5. However, corrections for multiple comparison resulted in no statistically significant relationships, demonstrating only weak and inconsistent evidence of the clinical benefits of continuity of care for women entering care for PTSD.
Grubaugh 2006[130]	Randomly identified female veterans who attended primary care clinic in any of the four VA sites in fiscal year 1999 (Charleston and Columbia, SC; Tuscaloosa and Birmingham, AL)	Females 187	Observational; To examine rates of medical and psychiatric disorders among female veterans, the recognition of such disorders by VAMC care providers, and the use of relevant medical and mental health services by women both within and outside of the VA setting	Frequency of psychiatric diagnoses, diagnostic accuracy, and medical comorbidity; Frequency of medical disorders and medical and psychiatric comorbidity; Functioning (SF-36 mental & physical health composite scores); Use of VA Health Services by psychiatric diagnosis; Use of outside care	Forty-four percent (43.9%) of women met criteria for at least one psychiatric disorder; 34.0% of these women met criteria for two or more additional psychiatric diagnoses, and concordance rates between interview and chart diagnoses were low. Ninety-five percent (95.2%) of women had a medical condition noted in their charts; 86.6% had two or more additional medical conditions, and a significant number of women had both medical and psychiatric diagnoses. Forty-four percent (43.9%) of women with an identified mental health condition received specialized mental health care by the VA in the past year.

Author	Sample Characteristics	Sample Size	Design/Objective	Main Measures	Main Findings
Gutierrez 2006[169]	Female and male soldiers who were processed for demobilization from military service between March 17, 2003 – November 3, 2003, through Fort Bliss, Texas	Females 897 Males 6386	Observational; To identify predictors of risky alcohol use and alcohol-related consequences among postdeployment soldiers	Prevalence of self-reported alcohol related consequences	Significant predictors of greater alcohol-related consequences, as assessed with the CAGE questionnaire, included fewer years of formal education, male, not being in an intimate relationship, racial/ethnic minority status, enlisted rank, having been deployed to the continental United States, and greater stress [$\chi^2(8,5,458) = 235.991$; $p < 0.001$]. Drinking and driving was more likely among soldiers who were male, not in a relationship, and reporting more stress than others in the sample [$\chi^2(8,5,384) = 50.241$; $p < 0.001$].
Halek 2005[142]	Female and male veterans who applied for posttraumatic stress disorder disability benefits.	Females 2466 Males 2452	Observational; To determine the incidence of spontaneously reported emotional distress caused by the survey and to see whether survey recipients experienced proximal increases in health care utilization relative to unsurveyed controls.	PTSD symptomatology, work, role, and social functioning, physical functioning, combat exposure and in-service sexual trauma, exposures to postservice traumas and hardships	Twenty-six percent of all surveyed veterans made a total of 1,542 spontaneous comments. The overall incidence of spontaneously reported emotional upset, however, was quite low, just 2.7% spontaneously reported experiencing emotional upset. Surveyed veterans spontaneously reporting emotional upset were more likely to be female and of American Indian or Native Alaskan race/ethnicity. They had more severe PTSD symptomatology and more exposures to postservice traumas and hardships; they were also substantially more likely than other respondents to say they had experienced an attempted or completed sexual assault while they were in the military. In general, both surveyed and unsurveyed veterans showed reduced outpatient health care use in the postsurvey period relative to the presurvey period.
Himmelfarb 2006[166]	Female veterans enrolled at a comprehensive women's program at the VA West Los Angeles Healthcare Center or invited by letter to participate in the study.	Females 196	Observational; To examine the prevalence and increased risk of posttraumatic stress disorder (PTSD) related to military sexual trauma (MST) and nonmilitary sexual trauma	Prevalence of sexual trauma; time period of sexual trauma and association with PTSD	Seventy-two percent of the sample had experienced sexual abuse. Military sexual trauma was significantly associated with PTSD (OR 4.30, 95%CI 2.30-8.00). The relative risk of participants with MST developing PTSD was almost 2 ½ times (RR=2.40) that of participants without MST. For those with postmilitary assault, the relative risk of developing PTSD was a little over 1 ½ times (RR=1.62) that of those without postmilitary assault. However, premilitary sexual assault (OR 3.52, 95%CI 1.64-7.57) and MST (OR 1.99, 95%CI 1.01-3.95) were each associated with post-military assault.

Author	Sample Characteristics	Sample Size	Design/Objective	Main Measures	Main Findings
Hoge 2007[13]	Female and male Iraq veterans, from four Army combat infantry brigades, surveyed 1 year after their return from deployment	80 Females 2783 Males	Observational; This study evaluated the association of PTSD with physical health measures among Iraq war veterans 1 year after their return from deployment with control for combat injury.	Past month symptoms of PTSD, depression, alcohol misuse, self-rated health status, sick call visits, missed work days, and somatic symptoms.	Among all participants, 16.6% met screening criteria for PTSD. PTSD was significantly associated with lower ratings of general health, more sick call visits, more missed workdays, more physical symptoms, and high somatic symptom severity. These results remained significant after controlling for being wounded or injured. The high prevalence of PTSD and its strong association with physical health problems among Iraq war veterans have important implications for delivery of medical services. The medical burden of PTSD includes physical health problems; combat veterans with serious somatic concerns should be evaluated for PTSD.
Kaplowitz 2006[34]	Female and male veterans at least 20 years old who had used outpatient services in the VA New England Health Care System at least once between January 1998 and December 1999 and at least once between January 2000 and June 2001	Females 2744 Males 61746	Observational; To examine the relationship between mental illness, health care utilization and rates of cholesterol testing	receipt of cholesterol testing; mental illness diagnosis; frequency of VA outpatient visits	Among veterans using VA outpatient services infrequently, those with mental illness were less likely than non-mentally ill control subjects to receive a cholesterol test during the study period (first quartile adjusted OR [aOR]=0.45, 95% CI 0.37–0.54; second quartile aOR=0.50, 95% CI 0.45–0.57). Mentally ill subjects with more frequent utilization of VA services were as likely as (third quartile aOR=1.01, 95% CI 0.91–1.13) or more likely than (fourth quartile aOR=2.73, 95% CI=2.46–3.03) non-mentally ill subjects to receive cholesterol testing. Mental illness was associated with a lower likelihood of cholesterol testing in subjects who used fewer VA outpatient services. The observed disparity attenuated at higher levels of service utilization.

Author	Sample Characteristics	Sample Size	Design/Objective	Main Measures	Main Findings
Kilbourne 2007[195]	Female and male veterans in VA National Psychosis Registry (NPR) database who also completed the VA's Large Veteran Health Survey of Veteran Enrollees (LHSV) subsection on health and nutrition behaviors.	Females 372	Observational; To evaluate patient and medication treatment factors associated with self-reported oral health status in patients diagnosed with serious mental illness (SMI) in a large, national sample of patients in the Veterans Affairs (VA) health System.	The study measured pre-disposing characteristics (race/ethnicity, education), enabling factors (unemployment, financial strain, smoking), treatment factors (use of tricyclic antidepressants or other medications) and oral health status (general oral health and dental problems that made it difficult to eat).	-Sixty-one percent of persons with SMI self-reported fair to poor dental health, 34.1 percent reported that oral health problems made it difficult for them to eat. -Patients who were not employed, experiencing financial strain, who smoked, who were prescribed tricyclic antidepressants, or prescribed selective serotonin reuptake inhibitors were more likely to report poor or fair dental health. These variables were also associated with having tooth or mouth problems.
Kimerling 2007[180]	Female and male veteran outpatients who were treated in VA health care settings nationwide during 2003.	Females 185880 Males 4139888	Observational; To examine (1) whether universal screening for military sexual trauma (MST) detects a substantial population of VHA patients who report MST, (2) whether a greater burden of medical and mental illness is found among patients who screen positive for MST compared with patients who screen negative, and (3) whether the burden of illness associated with MST varies by patient gender	MST brief screening instrument items, physical health diagnoses, and demographics	Screening was completed for 70% of patients. Positive screens were associated with greater odds of virtually all categories of mental health comorbidities, including posttraumatic stress disorder (adjusted odds ratio [AOR]=8.83; 99% confidence interval [CI]=8.34, 9.35 for women; AOR=3.00; 99% CI=2.89,3.12 for men). Significant gender differences emerged. The association of PTSD to MST was almost 3 times stronger among women than among men. The link between adjustment disorders and MST was significantly stronger among men than among women. Alcohol disorders and anxiety disorders were more common among both women and men who reported MST, but the relation to MST was significantly stronger among women than among men.
Lambert 2006[26]	Female and males forming a case series	1 Female 4 Males	Observational; To report a series of consecutive cases of PTSD affected combat veterans who were treated with the atypical antipsychotic agent aripiprazole (i.e., Abilify)	Sleep disturbances, nightmares, anxiety in crowds	The five cases combat-related PTSD treated with aripiprazole and either sertraline or cognitive-behavioral psychotherapy illustrate a significant improvement, but not total resolution of symptoms in most cases.

Author	Sample Characteristics	Sample Size	Design/Objective	Main Measures	Main Findings
Lande 2007[170]	Female and male participants were recruited from the Medical Center Brigade at WRAMC including two groups (1) clinical staff and (2) military patients.	Females 325 Males 685	Observational; To determine whether there are gender-based differences in alcohol use among US Army soldiers, and if so, to evaluate the role of alcohol education efforts in the military.	Alcohol consumption patterns both in terms of frequency and quantity, potential consequence experienced by subjects after alcohol consumption, awareness of and knowledge about alcohol, and level of interest in educational interventions and alcohol-free living areas	Although men were more likely to engage in "bolus" (binge) drinking, women exceeded established guidelines for safe alcohol consumption at a risk-adjusted rate nearly twice that of men. In addition, for individuals whose behaviors were not in conformity with public health guidelines for safe alcohol consumption, the severity of reported negative consequences was influenced by gender. Women initially experience greater psychosocial impairment, and—should harmful drinking patterns progress to alcohol dependency – they are at greater risk of injury, morbidity, and mortality than men.
Lang 2008[150]	Female VA primary care patients at San Diego VA	Females 221	Observational; To evaluate the relationships among childhood maltreatment, sexual trauma in adulthood, PTSD, and health functioning in women	PTSD and physical and mental health functioning	1. Childhood nonsexual maltreatment and adult sexual assault were positively associated with PTSD. 2. Childhood nonsexual maltreatment and PTSD were significantly associated with poorer physical and mental health functioning. 3. Adult sexual assault negatively affected health functioning through its association with PTSD.
Lang 2006[133]	Female veterans who received medical care from San Diego VA Healthcare System	Females 221	Observational; To examine whether current post-traumatic stress disorder (PTSD) mediates the relationship between exposure to childhood maltreatment (CM) and indicators of health and healthcare utilization in female veterans	Relationship between PTSD, exposure to childhood maltreatment (CM) and indicators of health and healthcare utilization	Increased emotional abuse ($\beta = -.32, p = .02$) was associated with poorer functioning on the SF-36 role-physical scale; increased emotional neglect ($\beta = .27, p = .02$) was associated with better functioning on the same scale. Higher levels of emotional abuse ($\beta = -.32, p = .01$) were associated with increased SF-36 bodily pain and greater odds of using pain medication in the past 6 months ($OR = 1.14, p = .01$). Greater physical abuse scores was associated with poorer SF-36 general health ($\beta = -.24, p = .04$), and CM was not associated with increased healthcare utilization. PTSD was shown to mediate the relationship between emotional and physical abuse and health outcomes.

Systematic Review of Women Veterans Health Research 2004-2008

Author	Sample Characteristics	Sample Size	Design/Objective	Main Measures	Main Findings
Lang 2005[55]	Female veterans who utilized the VA San Diego Healthcare System in 1998 at five different sites	Females 221	Observational; To examine the association between satisfaction with general medical services and trauma-related mental health symptoms in women.	overall satisfaction with visit; satisfaction with the provider; satisfaction with the clinic	The majority of patients were pleased with care they received. Older age and better mental health were significantly associated with greater overall satisfaction. The association between PTSD symptoms and satisfaction approached significance. Only general mental health reached significance individually with both satisfaction with the provider and the clinic. Women with more PTSD symptoms appear to be more satisfied with their overall care and with their provider.
Lapierre 2007[22]	Female and male active duty soldiers, who participated in a reintegration training program after returning from Iraq or Afghanistan	263 Females 3826 Males	Observational; To identify rates of posttraumatic stress and depressive symptoms in soldiers returning from war	Self-reported levels of depressions, posttraumatic stress, and life satisfaction	(1) Women comprised only a small sample (6%). (2) Shortly after deployment, about 44% of study participants reported clinically significant depressive and/or posttraumatic stress symptoms. Soldiers returning from Iraq reported somewhat more mental health problems and treatment seeking than soldiers returning from Afghanistan. (3) Being separated or divorced (vs. married) was associated with increased reports of posttraumatic stress and depressive symptoms. Compared to NCOs and officers, junior enlisted soldiers reported more posttraumatic and depressive symptoms. (4) Female participants were more likely to report depressive symptoms; however, gender was not a predictor for posttraumatic stress symptoms for either sample (OIF and OEF). (5) Soldiers seek help for the symptoms; however, only 16% of OIF participants and 13% of OEF participants with symptoms did so.
Lee 2007[182]	Female veteran convenience sample drawn from a pool of veterans who were participating in ongoing women's health and mental health research within a hospital setting.	Females 31	Observational; To understand how sexual trauma influences examination-related distress in female veterans, with the goal of improving the provision of care for this population.	Level of anxiety that women who had suffered sexual trauma experienced during breast, pelvic and rectal examinations, specifically relating to the gender of the provider. Prevalence of post traumatic stress disorder (PTSD) was also measured.	-The women reported significantly more anticipated anxiety during breast, pelvic, and rectal examinations when clinician gender was male (p<0.001 for each exam). Severity of PTSD symptoms was generally unrelated to anticipated examination-related anxiety, except for rectal exam. -Anticipated anxiety was found to be a function of both examination type and clinician gender but not of PTSD symptom severity. These findings emphasize the importance of screening for sexual trauma and the careful consideration of female veterans' unique needs during sensitive medical procedures.

Systematic Review of Women Veterans Health Research 2004-2008

Author	Sample Characteristics	Sample Size	Design/Objective	Main Measures	Main Findings
Mancino 2006[146]	Female and male veterans recruited from a 5-week, referral-based, VA outpatient psychosocial treatment program for PTSD from one site.	Females 5 Males 90	Observational; To evaluate the quality-adjusted health status in veterans with posttraumatic stress disorder (PTSD)	Association between symptom severity in veterans with PTSD and the quality-adjusted health status	The relationship between the QWB-SA and depression severity was linear (BDI quadratic, $p = 0.31$) and the linear relationship was significant ($p = 0.003$). The relationship between the QWB-SA and PTSD symptom severity as measured by the M-PTSD was linear (quadratic M-PTSD, $p = 0.33$), and the linear relationship was significant ($p = 0.02$). The relationship between the QWB-SA and the PTSD symptom severity as measured by the CAPS was nonlinear (CAPS quadratic term, $p < 0.05$). Overall, an inverse relationship was found between the quality of well being and PTSD and depression symptoms in Veterans. No findings reported by gender.
Merrill 2006[191]	Female and male US Navy recruits	Females 2321 Males 2435	Observational; To examine whether premilitary intimate partner violence (IPV) was associated with attrition	Military attrition based on 4 year follow-up in the Career History Archival Medical and Personnel System database of the Naval Health Research Center	Overall, more than one-fourth of recruits reported premilitary physical IPV and more than two-thirds reported premilitary verbal IPV. Women reported more perpetration and receipt of IPV than men, and married or cohabiting respondents reported more IPV than single respondents. Both perpetration and receipt of IPV significantly predicted attrition within 4 years. However, after controlling for other forms of IPV, only receipt of physical IPV significantly predicted attrition. In only one analysis did associations between IPV and attrition vary according to marital status or gender; premilitary receipt of verbal IPV had different effects on women and men.
Miller 2006[132]	National sample of female and male VA users during FY 2000 with no evidence of nursing home treatment during FY 1999 or FY 2000, followed through FY 2003 using administrative claims data.	Females 17096 Males 206760	Observational; To determine whether patients with mental health diagnoses in the Department of Veterans Affairs (VA) are more likely to be admitted to nursing homes and to identify sociodemographic, utilization, and clinical characteristics associated with nursing home admission	Relationship between number of diagnosed mental illnesses and the risk of being admitted to a nursing home	Among mentally ill patients, risk of admission was highest for those with any inpatient medical/surgical days (odds ratio [OR] 2.28, 95% confidence interval [CI] 2.13-2.43), followed by 3+ outpatient medical visits (OR 1.48, 95% CI 1.42-1.55), inpatient mental health days (OR 1.31, 95% CI 1.22-1.40), and outpatient mental health visits (OR 1.09, 95% CI 1.02-1.18). Patients diagnosed with dementia were 58% more likely to be admitted. Patients admitted to nursing homes were more likely to be older ($P < 0.0001$), men ($P < 0.0001$), white ($P < 0.0001$), single ($P < 0.0001$), had higher incomes ($P < 0.0001$), and suffered from greater service-related disability ($P < 0.0001$).

Author	Sample Characteristics	Sample Size	Design/Objective	Main Measures	Main Findings
Mojtabi 2003[138]	Female and male sample from National Collaborative Study of Early Psychosis and Suicide and comprised of U.S. Armed Forces personnel who had their first admission for major depression, bipolar disorder, or schizophrenia to a DoD hospital and were subsequently discharged from military services.	Females 754 Males 2106	Observational; To examine the use of Department of Veterans Affairs (VA) aftercare services among patients with serious mental disorders who were discharged from the military after a first admission to the Department of Defense (DoD) hospital.	Predictors of contact with VA versus no contact, and time to contact for those that do contact services.	Fifty-two percent of 2,861 identified individuals had received outpatient care from VA mental health clinics by the end of September 1998. Women, older persons, and persons with schizophrenia or bipolar disorder were more likely to contact VA outpatient mental health services than men, younger persons, and those with major depression. Also, being female, older than 25 years at military separation and having a diagnosis of bipolar disorder or schizophrenia were predictors of contacting services: women were more likely than men to use services.
Monnier 2004[151]	Female veterans identified from primary care clinics in four VA Medical Centers (Charleston and Columbia, SC; Tuscaloosa and Birmingham, AL).	Females 191	Observational; To examine the relationship between post tramatic stress disorder (PTSD) symptomatology, demographic variables, and functional status in US female veterans	Post tramatic stress disorder (PTSD) checklist (PCL)	After adjusting for other demographic covariates, PTSD severity was related to age (older patients reported less symptoms), and employment status (veterans who were not working due to disability reported significantly more PTSD symptoms than those who were working) for the female veterans. Additionally, after adjusting for relevant demographic covariates, greater PTSD symptomatology was related to worse functioning across both physical and mental health domains on the SF-36.
Murdoch 2007[181]	Female and male active duty Army and other service members	Females 327 Males 487	Observational; To describe functioning and psychiatric symptoms of active duty men and women stationed on U.S. soil who did and did not report experiencing military sexual stressors.	Sexual identity challenges measured using five items adapted from the gender role enforcement subscale of the Sexual Harassment of Men scale, sexual harassment, sexual assault	Forty-five percent of men and 80% of women reported at least one sexual stressor type (i.e., sexual identity challenges, sexual harassment, or sexual assault). After adjustment, subjects reporting more types of sexual stressors had poorer physical, work, role, and social functioning; more-severe post-traumatic stress disorder, depression, and anxiety symptoms; and more somatic concerns, compared with subjects reporting fewer or no sexual stressor types (all $p <0.004$). Interactions by gender were insignificant (all $p >0.11$). Within sexual stressor category, men and women reported similar mean adjusted functioning and psychiatric symptoms.

Author	Sample Characteristics	Sample Size	Design/Objective	Main Measures	Main Findings
Murdoch 2006[185]	Nationally representative sample of females and males seeking VA disability compensation (for PTSD) between 1994 and 1998	Females 1682 Males 1655	Observational; To describe the association between post-traumatic stress disorder (PTSD) and in-service sexual harassment in a nationally representative sample of Department of Veterans Affairs PTSD disability applicants	History of in-service sexual assault, combat exposure to serious postservice traumas and hardships, 3 items from sexual harassment inventory (SHI) criminal sexual misconduct subscale plus a fourth question about sexual assault unrelated to work	After adjustment for other reported traumas, women's reported in-service sexual harassment severity was significantly associated with PTSD symptom severity ($p < 0.0001$). The effect seen was about the same size as that seen for combat exposure among the men and for in-service sexual assault among the women. Men showed no association between in-service sexual harassment and PTSD ($p = 0.33$), although power was low for this test.
Murdoch 2005[157]	Nationally representative sample of disability benefit-seeking male and female veterans	Females 1682 Males 1655	Observational; To assess the impact of Veterans Affairs (VA) disability benefits for posttraumatic stress disorder (PTSD) on veterans' odds of poverty, especially in women and African Americans.	Receipts of VA disability benefits for PTSD or other, low income	Women were not significantly more likely than men to report low income. However, African Americans were more likely to report low income until adjustment for VA PTSD benefit was included.
Murdoch 2005[159]	Female and male representative, eligible veterans who file PTSD disability claims between 1994 and 1998.	Females 1678 Males 1653	Observational; To determine whether previously identified regional variations in PTSD disability awards are explained by appropriate subject characteristics (eg. differences in PTSD symptomatology or dysfunction) and to estimate the impact of veterans' PTSD symptom severity or level of dysfunction on their odds of obtaining PTSD disability benefits.	Rates of service connection for PTSD; PTSD symptom severity and functional status	Regional variation in PTSD disability awards could not be attributed to regional differences in veterans' current PTSD symptom severity or level of disability. PTSD symptom severity was associated with greater odds of service connection for PTSD ($P<0.0001$). Unexpectedly, poorer work, role, and social functioning and poorer physical functioning were each associated with lower odds of PTSD service connection ($P<0.0001$). Gender-specific data are only shown for the rates of service connection for PTSD by region.

Author	Sample Characteristics	Sample Size	Design/Objective	Main Measures	Main Findings
Murdoch 2004[188]	Nationally representative sample of females and males seeking VA disability compensation (for PTSD) between 1994 and 1998	Females 1683 Males 1654	Observational; To describe the prevalence of sexual assault among combat and noncombat veterans VA disability for posttraumatic stress disorder (PTSD).	Prevalence of sexual assault	In this study, approximately 4% of males and 63% of females with combat exposure experienced sexual assault in-service. For non-combat exposed veterans, approximately 13% of males and 75% of females experienced sexual assault in-service. For males, post-service sexual assault was greater than in-service, and for women in-service sexual assault was greater than post-service.
Murdoch 2003[158]	Randomly selected female and male veterans seeking VA disability benefits for PTSD between January 1994 and January 1998 who returned usable surveys	Females 1683 Males 1654	Observational; To see if there are gender discrepancies in rates of service connection for posttraumatic stress disorder (PTSD) and, if so, to see if these discrepancies could be attributed to appropriate subject characteristics (e.g., differences in symptom severity or impairment).	Gender-specific estimated rates of service connection for PTSD, unadjusted and adjusted for socio-demographic characteristics, PTSD severity/functional impairment, in-service sexual assault status, and combat exposure	A total of 3337 veterans returned usable surveys (effective response rate, 68%). Men's unadjusted rate of service connection for PTSD was 71%; women's, 52% ($P < 0.0001$). Adjustment for veterans' PTSD symptom severity or functional impairment did not appreciably reduce this discrepancy, but adjustment for dissimilar rates of combat exposure did. Estimated rates of service connection were 53% for men and 56% for women after adjusting for combat exposure.
Ouimette 2004[147]	Female and male patients in general medical and women's health clinics at the Department of Veterans Affairs Medical Center in Palo Alto and Menlo Park.	Females 82 Males 52	Observational; To examine the relationship between PTSD and health in medical patients within the Department of Veterans Affairs healthcare system, specifically among medical samples such PTSD patients with different etiologic traumas.	PTSD severity and diagnosis, mental health conditions (depressive disorder, panic disorder, generalized anxiety disorder), other medical diagnoses, health related quality of life (physical function, role limitations, pain, energy), health risk behaviors (weight, smoking, alcohol consumption), demographics.	-PTSD diagnosis and symptoms were associated with a higher likelihood of circulatory and musculoskeletal disorders. --PTSD symptoms were associated with more medical conditions. -PTSD symptoms and diagnoses were also associated with poorer health related quality of life. Most findings remained significant after controlling for comorbid mental health conditions. -Overall, gender did not moderate the relationship between PTSD and poorer health.

Systematic Review of Women Veterans Health Research 2004-2008

Author	Sample Characteristics	Sample Size	Design/Objective	Main Measures	Main Findings
Pierce 1998[178]	Female, Gulf War, Air Force veteran mothers of minor children	Females 263	Observational; To examine the predictors of children's adjustment problems in data collected from a representative sample of Air Force mothers two years after the Gulf War.	Strains in major life domains (job, financial, parenting, etc); mental health and well-being of mothers (depression, anxiety, etc); wartime life changes and adjustment problems of children (amount of time spent away from military parent, number of life changes, children's adjustment problems, etc.)	The deployment of military mothers during Desert Storm was shown to put children of those mothers at risk for various adjustment problems. These risks increased significantly when the mother was deployed in the theater of war, when she experienced difficulties in providing care for the children she left behind, and when her deployment resulted in significant changes in her children's lives.
Polusny 2008[124]	Female veterans completing an anonymous cross-sectional survey and enrolled in an outpatient VA clinic.	Females 456	Observational; To examine the difficulties Identifying one's emotions (alexithymia) in understanding the link between PTSD symptoms and negative health outcome in sexually victimized female veterans	Physical health complaints, VA urgent healthcare utilization, sexual trauma exposure (Traumatic Life Events Questionnaire; TLEQ), PTSD symptom severity, and alexythymia (Toronto Alexithymia Scale; TAS-II)	A total of 57.5% reported a lifetime history of sexual trauma; 45.8% reported sexual trauma before age 18; and 32.2% reported sexual trauma after age 18. Hierarchial regression analyses showed that alexithymia independently explained unique variance in participants physical health and their visits to urgent care. These data suggest that emotion recognition problems may contribute to poorer heath outcome in sexually traumatized women veterans beyond what is explained by sexual trauma exposure, health risk behaviors and PTSD. Psychological interventions that enhance emotion identification skills for women who have experienced sexual trauma could improve health perceptions and reduce need for acute health care.
Riddle 2007[175]	Female and male service members in a large US military cohort (the Millennium Cohort).	Females 20424 Males 56052	Observational; To describe the baseline prevalence of mental disorders in a large US military cohort	Baseline prevalence of mental disorders in a large US military cohort	(1) Alcohol abuse defined by PHQ was the most prevalent mental health disorder identified in the cohort. (2) The prevalence of all disorders was higher in women when compared with men except for alcohol abuse. Women were at statistically significant increased adjusted odds of PTSD, major depressive disorder, panic syndrome, anxiety syndrome, and eating disorders. (3) Generally, populations at greater odds of mental disorders included women, young, and single personnel, and individuals with lower socioeconomic status as measured by education enlisted rank, and length of service.

Author	Sample Characteristics	Sample Size	Design/Objective	Main Measures	Main Findings
Rowan 2006[140]	Female and male active duty Air Force Service Members seen in 8 outpatient mental health clinics during a 1-year period	Females 393 Males 812	Observational; To examine whether self-referred service members (SMs) are more likely to complete treatment than service members (SMs) referred by supervisors or those undergoing commander-directed evaluations.	Referral source (self, superiors encourages, commander directed), rank, special duty status, diagnostic category, treatment status, recommendations	Results showed significant differences across all variables, with self-referred members being more likely to be older, single, higher ranking, and without special duty status, as well as to have a less significant axis I diagnosis. Self-referred members were less likely to have confidentiality broken and to have career-affecting recommendations made. The implications of these findings, in terms of targeting interventions to increase self-initiated help-seeking behavior, and recommendations for future research are discussed.
Sadler 2004[190]	Female veterans who served in Vietnam and subsequent eras selected from comprehensive women's healthcare centers' registries at VA's in Boston, Durham, Tampa, Minneapolis, Chicago, and Los Angeles	Females 526	Observational; To determine whether the type or frequency of intentional violence experiences among women during military service influences health status or healthcare utilization. Differences in utilization and health status were also examined while controlling for life span violence exposures and important patient characteristic confounders.	Exposure to trauma, including sexual assault and military experiences, socio-demographics, current medical and mental health conditions and treatments, outpatient healthcare utilization, health status,	The type of violence women experienced was unrelated to differences in medical utilization. Women reporting repeated violence exposures during military service had significantly more outpatient visits in the year preceding the interview than singly or non-traumatized peers (16 vs. 9 and 8 visits, respectively, p ! 0.05). Repeatedly assaulted women also had poorer health status (p < 0.05), and more often reported a history of childhood violence (p ! 0.001) and post-military violence (p < 0.001). Repeated violence exposure is a relatively common experience among women in the military, and this has substantial implications for their health.
Sadler 2001[193]	National sample female veterans who served in Vietnam, post Vietnam or Persian Gulf War era and were in a VA registry	Females 537	Observational; To identify workplace factors associated with non-fatal physical assault occurring to women during military service, not in the context of rape or domestic violence.	Physical assault, sexual harassment, socio-demographic and environmental factors	Workplace violence was a common experience for military women. More than three-fourths of participants (79%) reported experiences of sexual harassment during their military service. Over half (54%) reported unwanted sexual contact. Threatened or completed physical assault was experienced by 36% of women during military service. In regression analyses, multiple risk factors increased the odds of physical assault from 3 to 7 fold including: experiencing unwanted sexual advances or pressure for dates in sleeping quarters (7fold); experiencing hostile work environments (5fold); observing heterosexual sexual activities in sleeping quarters (4fold); and ranking officers making sexually demeaning comments or behaviors (3fold).

Author	Sample Characteristics	Sample Size	Design/Objective	Main Measures	Main Findings
Sadler 2000[194]	National sample female veterans who served in Vietnam, post Vietnam or Persian Gulf War era and were in a VA registry	Females 537	Observational; To identify differences in health related quality of life among women veterans who were raped, physically assaulted, (not in the context of rape or domestic violence), both or neither during military service.	Health related quality of life scores	Nearly half (48%) the women experienced violence during military service, including rape (30%), physical assault (35%), or both (16%). Women who were raped or dually victimized were more likely to report chronic health problems, prescription medication for emotional problems, failure to complete college, and annual incomes less than $25,000 (p<.05) Those who had both traumas reported the most severe impairment, across all domains of health status.
Sajatovic 2006[196]	Female and male patients were recruited as part of VA Cooperative Study #430, Reducing the Efficacy-Effectiveness Gap in Bipolar Disorder, a randomized controlled trial that compared an easy-access treatment program and usual VA care.	Females 16 Males 168	Observational; To evaluate factors related to medication treatment adherence.	Factors associated with self reported treatment adherence among veterans with bipolar disorder such as patient characteristics, features of the patient-provider relationship, and barriers to care.	(1) Individuals with bipolar disorder who were non-adherent to medication were more likely to have current substance use disorder; alcohol was the most commonly abused substance. (2) Past substance use disorder does not appear to be associated with treatment non-adherence. (3) Individuals who were non-adherent to medication were less likely than those who were adherent to receive disability benefits. (4) Individuals who were adherent to medication had more prescriptions for different medications than those who were not adherent. No findings were reported by gender.
Schnurr 2008[154]	358 male Vietnam veterans who took part in a randomized clinical trial of group psychotherapy for PTSD and 203 female participants who took part in a randomized clinical trial of individual PTSD treatment, in Department of Veterans Affairs settings	Females 203 Males 358	Observational; To explore gender differences in quality of life among patients with post-traumatic stress disorder (PTSD)	Quality of life, PTSD symptoms	Overall quality of life was poor in men and women, and in general, they did not differ in quality of life or in how PTSD was associated with quality of life. The few statistically significant differences were small and clinically insignificant. For both men and women, numbing was uniquely associated with reduced quality of life.
Schnurr 2007[6]	Female veterans and active duty personnel from 12 sites (VA and non-VA)	Females 284	Randomized Clinical Trial; To evaluate random assignment to receive prolonged exposure versus present-centered therapy by standard protocol for 10 weeks	PTSD symptom severity	-Prolonged exposure was associated with greater reduction of PTSD symptoms -Prolonged exposure patients were more likely no longer meet PTSD diagnostic criteria

Author	Sample Characteristics	Sample Size	Design/Objective	Main Measures	Main Findings
Schultz 2006[186]	Female veterans random-ly selected from patients enrolled in 1 VAMC women's clinic who had 1 visit in past year, and community, convenience sample of civilian women from health and social organizations	Females 223	Observational; The purpose of the study was to investigate childhood sexual abuse (CSA), adult-hood sexual victimization (ASV), and adulthood sexual assault (ASA) experiences in a comparison sample of female military veterans and civilian community members.	Rates of each type of sexual victimization (CSA, ASV, and ASA).	Women veterans were significantly more likely than civilian women to report adult sexual assault [22%; $x^2(1, N = 220) = 15.985, p = 0.000$]. Although comparable rates of CSA and ASV were found across groups, veterans more frequently reported a history of sexual abuse by a parental figure, longer durations of CSA, and significantly greater severity of ASV than civilians.
Sherman 2005[136]	Sample veterans (and their female partners) who served in the Vietnam War, had a diagnosis of PTSD and service-connected disability for PTSD, par-ticipated in the PTSD program, and current cohabitation with a female partner recruited from two VA medical centers.	Females 72	Observational; To perform an initial needs assessment of partners of Vietnam veterans with combat-related post-tramatic stress disorder (PTSD) and to assess the partners' current rates of treatment use.	Partner treatment experienc-es and ratings of treatment needs; partners' assessment of her need for individual treatment and the partner's appraisal of family treatment being extremely important (yes/no).	Although large majorities of partners rated individual (64%) and family therapy (78%) to help cope with PTSD in the family as extremely or very important, only 28% had received any mental health care in the previous six months. Significant predictors of desire for individual treatment included partner's anxiety and patient-partner contact, and partner's age and severity of the patient's PTSD symptoms were signifi-cant predictors of family treatment. The most com-monly requested service was a women-only group.
Shipherd 2005[163]	Female and male Persian Gulf War military cohort returning from duty in 1991 and followed for 6 years	Females 102 Males 904	Observational; This study examined self-reported symptoms of PTSD and symptoms of drug and alcohol use (SUD) in a large non-treatment seeking popula-tion of veterans upon return from the Persian Gulf War and over a 6-year period to test the self-medication hypothesis.	Factors associated with substance use and PTSD symptoms	Those completing the survey at time T2 and T3 were more likely to be older, female, Caucasian, married, more educated, and a member of the Reserves or National Guard compared to non-completers. No dif-ference in substance use or PTSD symptoms occurred between completers and non-completers. A drug prob-lem at T2 prior to deployment and T2 PTSD arousal symptoms were predictive of T3 DAST scores, but these factors were not significant for MAST scores.

Author	Sample Characteristics	Sample Size	Design/Objective	Main Measures	Main Findings
Smith 2008[23]	Female and male active duty military enrolled in the Millenium Cohort Study surveyed before and after the wars in Iraq and Afghanistan	13849 Females 36279 Males	Observational; To investigate prospectively the effect of military deployment and self reported exposure to combat on new onset and persistent symptoms of PTSD in a large population based military cohort	Self-reported PTSD symptoms (PCL-C);	Over 40% of the cohort was deployed between 2001 and 2006; 24% deployed for the first time in support of the wars in Iraq and Afghanistan. Incidence rates of 10-13 cases of PTSD per 1000 person years occurred in the millennium cohort. New onset self reported PTSD symptoms or diagnosis were identified in 7.6-8.7% of deployers who reported combat exposures, 1.4-2.1% of deployers who did not report combat exposures, and 2.3-3.0% of nondeployers.
Smith 2008[10]	Female and male military service members previously deployed to Iraq and Afghanistan, exposed to combat, who had no PTSD at baseline assessment	Females 890 Males 4469	Observational; To conduct a prospective investigation of the relationship between prior assault and PTSD in a military cohort deployed to combat in Iraq and Afghanistan.	PTSD assessment, assault history, assault history, behavioral risk factors, and combat exposure .	-New-onset PTSD symptoms or diagnosis among deployed military reporting combat exposures occurred in 22% of women who reported prior assault and 10% not reporting prior assault. -Among men reporting prior assault, rates were 12% and 6%, respectively. -Adjusting for baseline factors, the odds of new-onset PTSD symptoms was more than 2-fold higher in both women and men who reported assault prior to deployment.
Stecker 2007[167]	VA national databases were used to identify veterans receiving IOP substance use treatment, and veterans with substance use disorders attending primary care but not in treatment	Females 247 Males 8082	Observational; To investigate gender differences among veterans receiving intensive outpatient (IOP) substance use treatment in a national VA sample and to compare women attending IOP with women with substance use disorders in VA primary care.	Psychiatric and medical conditions that co-occur with substance use disorder	Few women (2.8%) were treated in IOP at the VA. Among the women who did receive treatment, substantial clinical differences were found compared with men in IOP treatment. Women with substance use disorders were younger, more likely to have cocaine abuse or dependence disorders, and more likely to have extensive psychiatric and medical comorbidities than men with substance use disorders in the VA. Women in treatment were also found to be significantly different from women with substance use disorders not in treatment.

Author	Sample Characteristics	Sample Size	Design/Objective	Main Measures	Main Findings
Stein 2004[128]	Females in VA San Diego Healthcare System (VASDHS) primary care outpatient clinic.	Females 219	Observational; To determine whether there is an association between sexual assault history and measures of somatic symptoms and illness attitudes in a sample of female VA primary care patients, a group in whom high rates of sexual trauma have been reported.	Traumatic exposure, including sexual assault, physical complaints, healthcare utilization, reported sick days, somatization symptoms, health anxiety.	Sexual assault was associated with a significant increase in somatization scores, physical complaints across multiple symptom domains and health anxiety. Sexual assault was also a significant statistical predictor of having multiple sick days in the prior 6 months and of being a high utilizer of primary care visits in the prior 6 months.
Suris 2007[189]	Female veterans enrolled in a medical and/or mental health clinic in the VA North Texas Health Care System and had at least one outpatient visit in past 5 years	Females 270	Observational; To explore how differences in various assault types impact health outcomes.	Civilian sexual assault (CSA) and military sexual assault (MSA) histories, psychiatric symptoms, alcohol abuse, physical health functioning, quality of life	Women veterans with CSA histories reported significantly poorer physical, psychiatric, and quality-of-life functioning compared to those without a history of sexual assault. Women veterans with an MSA history demonstrated additional negative consequences above and beyond the effects of CSA.
Suris 2004[183]	Convenience sample of female veterans receiving medical and/or mental health treatment at the VA North Texas Healthcare System.	Females 270	Observational; To examine (1) the differential impact of military, civilian adult, and childhood sexual assault on the likelihood of developing posttraumatic stress disorder (PTSD); and (2) the relationship of military sexual assault (MSA) to service utilization and health care costs among women who access services through Veterans Affairs (VA).	Sexual assault history, PTSD, psychiatric diagnosis, utilization of care and care costs.	Compared with those without a history of sexual assault, female veterans were 9 times more likely to have PTSD if they had a history of MSA, 7 times more likely if they had childhood sexual assault (CSA) histories, and 5 times more likely if they had civilian sexual assault histories. An investigation of medical charts revealed that PTSD is diagnosed more often for women with a history of MSA than CSA. CSA was associated with a significant increase in health care utilization and cost for services, but there was no related increase in use or cost associated with MSA.

Author	Sample Characteristics	Sample Size	Design/Objective	Main Measures	Main Findings
Teh 2008[172]	Female and male VA patients in the National Psychosis Registry with a diagnosis of bipolar disorder, schizophrenia, schizoaffective disorder who completed the Large Health Survey of Veterans (LHSV) in FY 1999	Females 1324 Males 16693	Observational; To assess gender differences in health-related quality of life (HRQOL) in a national sample of veterans with serious mental illness (SMI)	Effect of gender on HRQOL (unadjusted and adjusted comparison), HRQOL of female and male veterans with SMI and female and male veterans without SMI, respectively (post hoc analysis to compare study results to normative data from previously published studies)	The sample was 7.3% female, 75.7% white, and 83.8% unemployed. Mean±SD age was 54.3±12.2 years. After the analysis adjusted for sociodemographic characteristics, health status, and other variables, compared with male veterans, female veterans with serious mental illness had lower scores on the SF-36 physical component summary (indicating worse symptoms), were more likely to report that they were limited "a lot" in activities of daily living, and had more pain. However, female respondents were more likely to have a positive outlook on their health.
Vinokur 1999[77]	Females in Air Force active duty reserve and guard forces.	Females 525	Observational; To examine the effects of work and family stressors and conflicts on Air Force women's mental health and functioning.	Job and parental stresses and work-family conflicts	Compared to the representative community sample, Air Force women had higher levels of family stress, work-family work conflicts, and job distress (p<0.05 for each measure).
Vogt 2008[145]	Female and male longitudinal cohort of active duty Marine Corp recruits at Parris Island surveyed at two time points	Females 678 Males 893	Observational; To examine the relationship between stress reactions and hardiness by gender during Marine Corp recruit training, and to examine how stress and hardiness differ based on social support.	Ratings of reactions to different stress factors, 3 domains of hardiness (i.e., control, commitment, and challenge); perceptions of social support, and negative emotions expressed	Women reported slightly higher levels of both negative affectivity (22.24 vs. 20.67) and stress reactions (21.93 vs. 19.52; p<.05 for each) at T1 compared with men. Women also reported slightly higher levels of stress reactions (19.01 vs. 16.34) and perceived social support (41.23 vs. 40.15; p<.05 for each) at T2 compared with men. Identified intercorrelations were similar across gender (e.g., negative affectivity had moderate relationships with both stress reactions and hardiness for both men and women, etc). Although the negative impact of stress reactions on hardiness was strongest when social support was low for both genders, stress reactions predicted enhanced hardiness when social support was high for women only.

Author	Sample Characteristics	Sample Size	Design/Objective	Main Measures	Main Findings
Vogt 2008[143]	National sample of female and male Gulf War I veterans	Females 80 Males 231	Observational; To identify differences in exposure to deployment stressors based on military status (i.e., active duty vs. National Guard/Reserve [NG/R] units) and to identify associations between deployment stressors and posttraumatic stress symptoms.	Deployment stressor scales (combat experiences, perceived threat, etc); predictors of posttraumatic stress symptomatology (PTSS)	-Active duty reported more significant combat experiences than NG/R personnel. The NG/R personnel reported more concerns about family/relationship disruptions than active duty. Deployment risk factors were positively associated with PTSS and resilience factors were negatively associated with PTSS. -The gender analysis indicated that perceived threat had greater PTSS associations for NG/R males compared to active duty males, while perceived threat had greater PTSS associations for active duty females compared to NG/R units.
Wallace 2006[173]	Random sample of female and male veteran enrollees who had used VHA services within the prior three years or who had enrolled in VHA in anticipation of using services in the future.	Total 128352 Female/ Male not listed	Observational; To study whether rural and urban disparities in health-related quality of life persist among veterans with common psychiatric disorders.	Health-related quality of life scores in rural and urban veterans with common psychiatric disorders.	(1) All psychiatric disorders except anxiety disorders not related to PTSD were more prevalent in urban groups. (2) Rural veterans within mental illness cohorts had worse PCS and MCS scores, denoting worse physical and mental health-related quality of life. (3) In regression models, rural-urban disparities within psychiatric disorder cohorts persisted after socio-demographic factors were controlled. No findings were reported by gender.
Westrup 2005[144]	Case study of 1 female veteran, who entered a residential program for treatment of PTSD	Females 1	Observational; Case study of the application of a non-traditional treatment (self defense training) for PTSD to treat the negative symptoms of PTSD.	Quality of life, personal safety and risk-taking	1) Physical skills training was empowering for the patient. 2) Didactic portion was illustrative of social psychological deficits that arise among women with trauma (e.g., not locking doors to car or house). Lessons targeted key skill deficits and faulty core beliefs (e.g., she brought trauma on herself). 3) Upon graduating from self-defense, she said she felt like she got her life back. The 6-month follow-up showed significant life changes: discarded weapons; bolstered home security; and beginning to socialize and travel again.

Author	Sample Characteristics	Sample Size	Design/Objective	Main Measures	Main Findings
Wolfe 2005[187]	Female and male US Marine Corp recruits at Parris Island	Females 698 Males 832	Observational; To study the impact of pre-military interpersonal trauma on attrition during USMC recruit training	Rates of interpersonal trauma by gender, time to attrition by gender, association of pre-military trauma and attrition	At least one type of trauma was reported by 47.5% of male recruits and 68.1% of female recruits (p<.01). Female recruits were more likely to be discharged compared with male recruits (HR 1.647, 95% CI 1.239 – 2.189). While retention rates for male recruits with and without a trauma history showed no difference, retention rates for female recruits with and without a trauma history significantly differed; females with an interpersonal trauma history were more likely to be discharged (HR 1.58, 95%CI 1.034 – 2.413).
Yaeger 2006[165]	Female veteran convenience sample in 1 VAMC comprehensive women's clinic	Females 196	Observational; To compare impact of military sexual trauma (MST) versus all other traumas on the rate of current PTSD diagnoses.	Rates of PTSD	In this group, 92% of women had at least 1 trauma; 41% had MST with or without other trauma; 90% had other trauma alone or in combination with MST. Moreover, 60% of those with MST and 43% of those with other trauma had PTSD. In logistic regression analyses, MST was a significant predictor of PTSD (OR 4.4, 95%CI 2.4, 8.2) and prior trauma was not (OR 1.3, 95%CI 0.63, 2.5).
Zeber 2007[105]	Female and male veterans in National Psychoses Registry from June 1, 2000, through September 30, 2003, for all veterans diagnosed with schizophrenia and receiving healthcare through the Department of Veterans Affairs.	Females 4275 Males 76393	Observational; To assess the effect of the 200 Veterans Millennium Health Care Act, which raised pharmacy copayments from $2 to $7 for lower-priority patients, on medication refill decisions and health services utilization among vulnerable veterans with schizophrenia.	Total prescription fills, medical and psychotropic fills separately, outpatient visits, psychiatric admission, inpatient days among those admitted, and pharmacy costs	Total prescriptions and overall pharmacy costs leveled among veterans with copayments after the medication cost increase. However, psychiatric drug refills dropped substantially, nearly 25%. Although outpatient visits were unaffected, psychiatric admissions and total inpatient days increased slightly, particularly 10-20 months after the policy change.

Author	Sample Characteristics	Sample Size	Design/Objective	Main Measures	Main Findings
Zivin 2007[199]	Female and male patients from the VA's National Registry for Depression (NARDEP) linked to data from the VA Medicare Data Merge Initiative and the National Death Index.	Females 46 Males 1637	Observational; To report clinical and demo-graphic factors associated with suicide among depressed veterans in an attempt to determine what characteristics identified depressed veterans at high risk for suicide.	Suicide and time until suicide	Increased suicide risks were observed among male, younger, and non-Hispanic White patients. Veterans without service-connected disabilities, with inpa-tient psychiatric hospitalizations in the year prior to their qualifying depression diagnosis, with comorbid substance use, and living in the southern or western United States were also at higher risk. Posttraumatic stress disorder (PTSD) with comorbid depression was associated with lower suicide rates, and younger depressed veterans with PTSD had a higher suicide rate than did older depressed veterans with PTSD. The relative risk ratio for men compared with women in the depressed VA population was somewhat smaller than that reported for the general population.

APPENDIX 10. PEER REVIEW COMMENTS

Reviewer	Comment	Change
LAB	I noted three articles that may have been missed in your review: (1) Vernon SW, del Junco DJ, Tiro JT, Coan SP, Perz CA, Bastian LA, Rakowski W, Chan W, Lairson DR, McQueen A, Fernandez ME, Warrick C, Halder A, DiClemente C. Promoting regular mammography screening II. Results from a randomized trial in US Women Veterans. J NCI 2008;100:347-358; (2) McQueen A, Swank PR, Bastian LA, Vernon SW. Predictors of perceived susceptibility of breast cancer and changes over time; a mixed modeling approach. Health Psych 2008;27:68-77; (3) Chireau MV, Salz T, Brown H, Bastian L. Outcomes, Costs, and Utilization of Pregnancy-related care. Federal Practitioner September 2006: 20-30. The most important article is by Vernon et al (pdf attached to Email). It is the companion article to Del Junco ref #83 (described on page 25) and presents results of a large NIH-funded trial designed to improve mammography adherence. I think it should be listed as an important clinical trial. The other 2 articles (are also attached) include an assessment of breast cancer risk perception among women veterans and a pilot study of pregnancy outcomes among women veterans using the VA.	We agreed with the recommendations and have added these 3 articles to the review.
LH	I have struggled with the formatting/organization. I recommend changing your fonts to more explicitly help the reader stay on track with the section they are reading. It might help to have more subsections. I struggled with having all of the ptsd/mental health stuff in the deployment section. It seems to me you need a clear cut mental health section and that those studies should be located there. Also, in general, I think the deployment/post-deployment section is very difficult to read and confusing. A clearer cut font font pattern might help with this.	We changed the size and font for the headers of each section and subsection to guide the reader more clearly through the report
LH	It is my view that there is too much reporting and too little synthesis in this report. I do not know the end user for this but if I were reading it or trying to use it for something what I would want is the bibliography at the end, perhaps organized more as I suggest above (more subcategories), with more synthesis in the text—really, kind of an expanded summary section. As an example, on page 26 there is a paragraph summarizing data on cvd risks. It might be more useful to expand this summary statement and note how little data there really are about cvd rf in women vets. I am struck by how little meaningful research has been done.	1) Due to the descriptive nature of literature covering a population and not a disease, some of this synthesis technique is limited. 2) We expanded the CVD summary comments to inform the reader of the limited nature of the data. 3) We are also creating an online database of these articles, as well as those from the previous report, that may act as an interactive searchable bibliography.
LH	Brainstorming, the organizational structure that makes sense to me is as follows: a. Mental health—ptsd, substance abuse, mst; b. Access; c. Gender specific health care—reproductive, breast, etc; d. Quality of care; e. Deployment/post-deployment care; f. Health care delivery; g. Utilization; h. Health care outcomes/ research; i. Maybe a specific oif/oef section. However, this is just brainstorming and I certainly don't know the ltierature well enough to feel any confidence about this. Again-rather than just reporting the results line by line, it seems to me this report needs the synthesis. It wouldn't matter to me if the paper was short if it provided meaningful summaries. You have all the data in the appendix.	Recommendations appreciated. Our general categories overlap with your suggestion. We plan to keep post-deployment and OEF/OIF sections separate from gen categories due to its special relevance with current veterans.
LH	I would add article titles and author names and maybe even the journal to the appendix tables 5-9 so readers can quickly figure out if they want to bother reading the results.	The current format is standard reporting style; the tables would be unwieldy otherwise.

141

PPS	Comprehensiveness: Last time, I had searched the PILOTS database on www.ptsd.va.gov to help out. PILOTS includes Medline, PsychInfo, and other databases and grey literatures, and indexes content according to a trauma-specific controlled vocabulary. For example, I believe the following articles I found thru PILOTS (quickly using the descriptors DE=female and (military personnel or veterans)) would be relevant but are not included. (1) An examination of family adjustment among Operation Desert Storm veterans Taft, Casey T; Schumm, Jeremiah A; Panuzio, Jillian; Proctor, Susan P Journal of Consulting and Clinical Psychology, vol. 76, no. 4, pp. 648-656, August 2008. (2) Alcohol use and alcohol-related problems before and after military combat deployment. Jacobson, Isabel G; Ryan, Margaret A K; Hooper, Tomoko I; Smith, Tyler Clain; Amoroso, Paul J; Boyko, Edward J; Gackstetter, Gary Dean; Wells, Timothy S; Bell, Nicole S. Journal of the American Medical Association, vol. 300, no. 6, pp. 663-675, August 13, 2008 And even PILOTS is not good enough, e.g., I found the following on PubMed (but not PILOTS) and would think it needs to be included: Distress and pain during pelvic examinations: effect of sexual violence. Weitlauf JC, Finney JW, Ruzek JI, Lee TT, Thrailkill A, Jones S, Frayne SM. Obstet Gynecol. 2008 Dec;112(6):1343-50.PMID: 19037045 [PubMed - indexed for MEDLINE] Maybe you found some of the articles I'm mentioning and decided to exclude them. If so, then I don't think the inclusion/exclusion criteria are correct because I don't see why you would not include a study on sexual trauma and pelvic exams in women	The articles located in the PILOTS database occurred at the end or after the search was completed in August 2008. They will be included in the next update to follow this one.
PPS	Timeliness: I think the report should be more current than 2008 because so much literature has emerged since 2008, particularly on younger veterans and service members, but also on older cohorts who are using VA in greater numbers. For example, in the quick search above (which probably should be expanded—our information scientist could advise you on the best way to do a comprehensive search for this topic), I found 31 articles 2004-2008 and 18 from 2009 to the present. I know the decision of where to cut is hard—we're currently dealing with this in a meta-analysis—but at the end of 2010 I would think this should be current at least thru 2009.	We agree with your suggestion. A subsequent update will follow this one for additional literature review.
PPS	Topics: It seems like aging is not addressed much in the literature, even though this is an issue for VA; more broadly, there is very little known about trauma in older women. Should this maybe mentioned? I may have missed it.	Very few articles covered aging veterans beyond the studies on medications in patients >65. We will add this area as a current gap to our report.
PPS	I also wondered if there is a meta-issue worth mentioning, which is that people sometimes do not report data on women separately even when they could.	Yes, some articles had data analyses with results by gender but did not report on it. Gender was often used as a control variable in large sample analyses. This finding is now listed within the body of the report.
AGS	There is a difference in presentation style in the deployment section in that authors names are not noted whereas in subsequent sessions they are done when possible. This might be due to multiple authors cited in some cases.	We corrected this error and included author names in the deployment section.

	Comment	Response
AGS	It would have been useful for the investigators to have used the (Appendix 1) screening form to comment within the text on the topics that did not meet with inclusion criteria and are deficits in our knowledge base or literature. For example, TBI or polytrauma work does not have a body of work that will benefit our understanding and care of women and I would also consider this as one of the ongoing gaps as well as the ones already identified (that are definitely on target). In short, including what isn't done using this thorough screener is also as important as what is done and summarized. However, given how well done this is, perhaps this might be considered in a brief summary paragraph and be sufficient. Another example of what is missing is literature on cervical cancer (Pap smear) screening compliance in women veterans and so forth.	We have added your suggestions (TBI, poly trauma data by gender, invasive exams among veteran women or women w trauma) to a current gaps in the literature section for the report.
SF	P6, Methods, criterion A: "(a) included women veterans,…" So, if a study included WV but did not specifically examine gender effects, was the study included?	Yes, a study was included if it included women vets but was not specifically done to examine gender effects.
SF	P6, Methods, criterion C: "(c) relevant to VA healthcare or how VA care is delivered to women…": First, do you mean, "relevant to VA women's healthcare?" Second, it seems like both clauses are talking about health care delivery, but I'm wondering if the first clause is supposed to be about health rather than delivery? Should it say, "relevant to women veterans' health or how VA care is delivered to women"?	Yes, we modified the phrasing using your suggestions.
SF	P7, Conclusions: I'm thinking you may be able to add a couple good "soundbites" in bold or italics, which may subsequently be picked up by the press or policymakers when they are referring to your report. For example, at the end of the first paragraph of conclusions: "Therefore, more women veterans health articles have been published in the past 5 years than in all of the 23 years before that." At the end of the last paragraph, "Therefore, the past 5 years have seen substantial alignment between priority areas for women veterans health research and the topic areas being pursued."	Thank you! These soundbite statements were added to the report with bold font.
SF	P8, PA1: does 44% refer to users or enrollees?	Corrected, enrollees.
SF	P9, PA1: did you use "military" (or equivalent) at all in the search strategy?	Did not use "military". Only used "Veterans".
SF	P13 Box showing 295 rejected, 151 abstract/title rejections: could potentially show the breakdown the same way you do in the lower box of 185 rejected (ie why the abstract/title was rejected)	Title and abstract rejections were done by team consensus in a meeting. The other rejections were decided using the formal screen and for a specific reason using 2 physician reviewers.
SF	P16 PA1: change "complete routine screening" to "complete routine gynecological screening"	Corrected.
SF	P17 PA4: I think the sentence could be inverted so the finding comes before the interpretation: "A key finding is that psychiatric diagnoses were common for both OEF and OIF evacuations, suggesting the need for DOD and VA to…"	Corrected.
SF	P20 PA1: Is a comma missing after "inpatient quality"?	Corrected.
SF	P21 PA1 (last line): should "perceptions" be "expectations"?	Yes, corrected.
SF	P25 PA1: I don't understand this sentence ("abstain or say no to sex" shows up twice in the sentence, and I don't understand what "compared to" means here.)	
SF	P25 PA4: This mentions a "mammogram intervention"; it would be nice to have a few words re what kind of intervention.	1 sentence explanation added.
SF	P26 PA2: Same thing, would be nice to have a few words describing the employee intervention.	1 sentence explanation added.

	Comment	Response
SF	P26 PA5: Refers to "sexual trauma patients" and "mental health/PTSD patients." Would avoid this terminology throughout—I imagine that some patients may read the report, and may be more comfortable with terminology like, "patients with a history of sexual trauma", "patients with mental illness [or mental health conditions]" etc.	Corrected phrasing as suggested.
SF	P31 PA3: "prevalence of violence" should be "prevalence of prior exposure to violence"	Corrected phrasing.
SF	P35 PA2: refers to "VA's first women's health research agenda" without explaining what this is.	First women's health research agenda is now explained.
SF	P35 PA4: Says that topic areas map to VA priorities. One idea for an appendix could be to list published VA priority areas and then map studies to them. Probably too involved at this late stage of report preparation, but could be something to consider for future.	Will consider adding this appendix piece to next update.
SF	P36 PA4: After the end of the sentence "subgroup analyses of women in VA" could add, "and demonstrates that it is feasible to conduct robust clinical trials in women veterans"	Corrected. Info added.
SF	P36 PA5: This mentions step 4 in the VA QUERI model; this comes a bit out of nowhere; consider including the QUERI model as an appendix? Again, probably too involved at this late stage, but in a future report it could be interesting to map studies to the QUERI model.	QUERI model reference was removed from this section.
SF	P36 PA6: I think the word "not" is missing, i.e., "VA studies have NOT yet made their mark…"	Corrected. "not" added.
SF	P36 PA7: I think point #1 should be preceded by the word "limited" and could also talk about combos of diseases, e.g., "Limited clinical and intervention outcome data for chronic physical or mental health conditions and complex combinations of diseases". In addition to these three points, would you also want to comment on the need for info about the impact of new re-design efforts (PCMH, WCHIP)?	Corrected. "limited" added.
SF	References: I notice that a few are from pre-2004 (eg references 35, 77). Is that intentional?	If articles from prior years were sent to us from VA investigators or from culling other citations, we included them in order to be as comprehensive as possible.
SF	When you mention odds ratios, could indicate whether they are adjusted (which could be done compactly by using the abbreviation AOR).	We changed ORs to AOR's where appropriate.
SF	Something to consider for the next time you do this is whether to also include methodological studies as a category. Hopefully some people will be publishing on what it takes to do women's health research in VA.	We will keep this consideration in mind for the next women vet lit update.
SF	Another thing to consider for the future would be whether to include the Impact Factor of journals in the table showing all articles. I have mixed feelings about this, because there are questions about how these impact factors are calculated. But, the reason I raise it is because there had been concern about whether research on women veterans is appearing in less visible journals, and it could be interesting to know whether this is starting to improve.	We decided not to include the impact factor of the journal to avoid the politics of publications.
SF	I notice that in some places in the document, important limitations of a study are mentioned, along with the findings. I thought they way you did that was effective. If anything, I would like to see that even more (or even having a limitations column in the Table), because of the concern that people who read this will cite conclusions of studies without understanding the caveats. However, in addition to being more work than is feasible at this point, that would make the report long and cumbersome. One idea might be to comment briefly on this issue early in the document, i.e., that each study has to be interpreted subject to limitations and it is not feasible to include all the caveats and limitations in this document, so before citing the findings the reader should refer to the source article.	We decided to briefly comment on this issue in the report. It is now included in the methods/results section.